REVERSE SKIN AGING

Using Your Skin's Natural Power

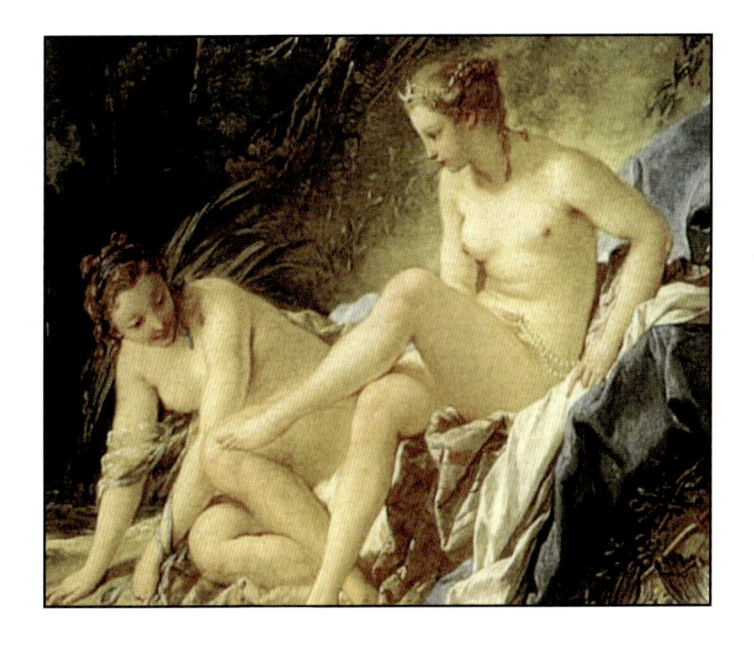

Loren Pickart, PhD
The Turn Back the Clock Doc

Disclaimer and Cautions

The ideas, procedures, and suggestions contained in this book are intended to help improve health and are not intended to act as a substitute for regular medical care by a qualified health-care professional. Some individuals may have success with skin products not mentioned in this book. Skin Biology products are designed to improve skin health, but should not be used on broken or wounded skin. All products applied to the skin should be started cautiously since individuals may have unique allergies or sensitivities. If you develop sensitivity to any skin-care or hair-care product, discontinue its use immediately and consult your physician. If skin problems persist or worsen, consult a physician. Neither the author nor the publisher will be responsible for any loss, injury, or damage arising from any information or suggestion in this book. None of the statements in this book have been approved by the FDA.

Copyright July 2005 by Loren Pickart.

Published by
Cape San Juan Press
Summit Associates International
12833 SE 40th Place
Bellevue, WA 98006
425-644-0160
www.skinbiology.com

FIRST PRINTING – JULY 2005.
ISBN 0-9771853-0-3

This book, or parts thereof, may not be reproduced in any form without written permission except for inclusion of quotations in a review.

These products are trademarks of the following companies: Neova, Tricomin, Graftcyte (Procyte Corporation); Active Copper, Visibly Firm, Retin-A, Renova (Johnson & Johnson); Propecia (Merck Corporation); Rogaine (Pharmacia & Upjohn Consumer Healthcare).

*In memory of my mother,
Grace Pickart,
who started all of this long ago
by taking me to see dinosaurs at museums....*

Table of Contents

CHAPTER ONE
Reverse Skin Aging: The Fountain of Youth   7
What is Reverse Aging?

CHAPTER TWO
Artificial and Unnatural Skin Treatments   12
Alien Chemicals, Junk Science, Cinderella Becomes Count Dracula
Unnatural and Artificial Methods of Skin Renewal

CHAPTER THREE
Remodeling – The Key to Youthful Skin   19
Why Do Children Have Such Beautiful Skin?
The Holy Grail of Skin Care
Maximizing the Skin's Natural Renewal Systems
The GHK-Cu Breakthrough – SRCPs Really Work!

CHAPTER FOUR
Using Second-Generation SRCPs   32
Tips for Natural Skin Renewal
My Approach to Making Skin Products

CHAPTER FIVE
Why Wrinkles Develop and How to Remove Them   39
Your Body's Natural Wrinkle Removal System
Types of Wrinkles
Testimonials & Experiences

CHAPTER SIX
Tighten Loose and Sagging Skin   53
The Benefits of Biological Skin Tightening
The Natural Way to Tighten Skin
Tightening Pores & Testimonials

CHAPTER SEVEN
The Balancing Act for Removing Scars and Blemishes   62
How to Reduce Acne Scars and Other Blemishes and
Help Your Skin Heal after Deep Peels, Laser Resurfacing, and Dermabrasion
Reduction of Skin Tags, Stretch Marks, Sun Damage, and Moles
Post-Procedure Healing

CHAPTER EIGHT
Special Concerns   75
When Make-up Ravages the Skin for Models, Actors and Make-up Lovers

CHAPTER NINE
SRCP Products for Improving Health of Extra-Sensitive Skin   79
BioHeal and CP Serum for "At Risk Skin"
Treating Eczema, Very Dry Skin, Diabetic Skin Problems, Burns, Allergies,
Dermatitis, Psoriasis, and other skin conditions...

CHAPTER TEN
Keeping Your Skin Young & Beautiful   89
The Protective Skin Barrier
Protecting Your Delicate Skin
Biological Healing Oils – Methods of Skin Moisturization

Chapter Eleven
Improving Hair Growth and Condition with SRCPs 101
Why the Big Apple is a Bad Hair Town
Hair Thinning and Loss
Using SRCPs to Stimulate Hair Growth — Hair Growth Recommendations

Chapter Twelve
Biology, Chemistry, and Hair Care 111
What Is Hair?
Factors that Damage Hair
Choosing the Right Shampoo & Conditioner
Permanents and Chemical Hair Relaxers
Longer Eyelashes, Thicker Eyebrows

Chapter Thirteen
The Formula of Love 124
The Two Types of Pheromones
Smells Affect Our Emotions
Efforts to Create an Effective Perfume — From Theory to Practice

Chapter Fourteen
Glowing Good Health 135
Better Suntanning with Less Skin Damage
Sunlight and Good Health
Chemical Sunscreens Aren't the Answer

Chapter Fifteen
Feeding Your Face and Body Nutrients that Turn Back the Clock 143
50,000 Years of Dietary Changes
Is the Recommended Daily Allowance Enough?
Supplements & Vitamins Recommended by Many Anti-Aging Scientists
Red Wine and Your Health

Chapter Sixteen
The Science Behind SRCPs 154
Experiments on Aging Reversal
Mechanism of Skin Repair and Remodeling
Second-Generation SRCPs — The Future of GHK-Cu

Chapter Seventeen
Copper: Your Body's Protective Anti-Aging Metal 168
The Two Forms of Copper
How Much Copper Do You Need?
Copper and Love — Ancient Ideas Rise Again

Chapter Eighteen
The Moral Need for Beauty 176
Cosmetics, Jewelry, Technology, Art, Symbolism
It's In Your Genes
The Power of Human Beauty

Chapter Nineteen
Resources 182

Chapter Twenty
References 187
Index of Words 193

— Your Special Offer —
Special Introductory Offer

Foreword and Acknowledgments

This book started more than 40 years ago with my rather naive idea of finding a way to reverse human aging. Over the years, this quest led me to laboratories in Minneapolis, Santa Barbara, San Francisco, Seattle, and finally to my home on San Juan Island where I am writing today. During the course of this journey, I was more successful than I had ever imagined in finding a human molecule that helps reverse many types of aging damage, which today is used in many cosmetic and dermatological products. But it took me until 2004 to truly understand how the body's aging reversal system works. This book details my findings.

The topics explored on the following pages arose from the thousands of questions I have received from Skin Biology clients. Most of these individuals were primarily interested in obtaining healthier, more beautiful skin and hair. But clients have also asked me about subjects such as pheromones, diets, supplements, suntanning, and the actual published science behind Skin Remodeling Copper Peptides (SRCPs), the skin's natural renewal signals. If you would like to quickly learn the best ways to benefit from SRCPs, read Chapters 3-9 and 11, which were written as "how-to" chapters.

I would like to thank those who helped me make this book a reality: Jennifer Schaefer for integrating and editing to produce a more understandable manuscript; Anna Margolina for suggestions and reviewing technical points for accuracy; Idelle Musiek for adding additional commentary that helped to bridge the gap between pedantic science and emotions (such as the thoughts that arise while sitting at a vanity table applying lip plumper); Enid Becker Smith, who drew the Garden of Eden and Breast Lift graphics, and The Bellevue Club of Bellevue, Washington for permission to use the "Turn Back the Clock Doc" graphic.

And a special thanks to Cassia McClain who expertly formatted the manuscript and illustrated most of the graphics within the book.

I also would like to thank all of the scientists, clinicians, and veterinarians around the world whose work finally enabled a biochemical understanding of the mode of action of remodeling copper peptides.

Finally, a big thanks to my daughters Francoise, Genevieve, Celine, and Lavinia for their comments, and to my beautiful, gracious, and talented wife Charlene for all her help and support.

> "Age seizes my skin and turns my hair from black to white; My knees no longer bear me and I am unable to dance like a fawn. What could I do? I am not ageless; My youth is gone. Red-robed Dawn, immortal goddess, carried Tithonus to earth's end. Yet age seized him despite the gift from his immortal lover... I love delicate softness; For me, love has brought the brightness and the beauty of the sun."
> – Sappho, fragment 58

Chapter 1

REVERSE AGING: The Fountain of Youth

Ancient alchemists had three goals: turning base metals into gold, flying to the moon, and finding the elixir of eternal life. The first two have been accomplished: lead can be turned into gold with an atomic accelerator and the moon bears human footprints. At long last, the final goal is becoming a reality, as biochemical discoveries are successfully reversing many of the harmful changes that occur in the body as the years pass.

As those over age 35 are well aware, time takes a toll on our skin. As we age, the skin becomes thinner and accumulates imperfections. The structural proteins are progressively damaged, causing collagen and elastin to lose resiliency. The skin's water-holding proteins and sugars diminish, the dermis and epidermis thin, the microcirculation becomes disorganized, and the subcutaneous fat cells diminish in number. Decades of exposure to ultraviolet rays, irritants, allergens, and various environmental toxins further intensify these effects. The result is wrinkled, dry, inelastic skin populated by unsightly lesions. See Figure 1.1

But you don't have to watch your skin's youthful look fade without a fight. This book reveals practical ways to reverse the harmful effects of aging, and in many cases how to stop these effects before they occur. Most of the methods on the following pages are based on my research that led to the discovery of Skin Remodeling Copper Peptides, or SRCPs – a signal in the body that helps trigger the skin's natural mechanism of renewal, restoring the skin to a biologically younger and healthier condition. Later chapters discuss how to reverse the effects of aging on other regions of the body, such as the scalp and its hair.

Oily: 15% of skin lipids are squalane/squalene

Skin is smooth and blemish free

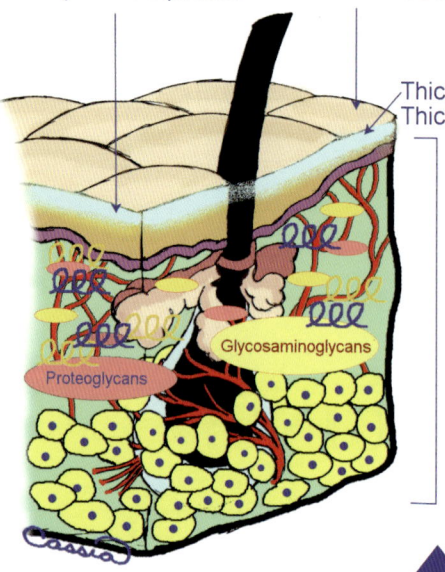

Thick acid mantle
Thick skin depth

Glycosaminoglycans

Proteoglycans

Young Skin

Dense capillary beds, undamaged collagen and elastin, ample water-holding proteins, plus a thick layer of subcutaneous fat, large follicles, and adequate stem cells

lll : collagen
lll : elastin

Aging

Aging Reversal

Skin is wrinkled and inelastic

Dry: 5% of skin lipids are squalane/squalene

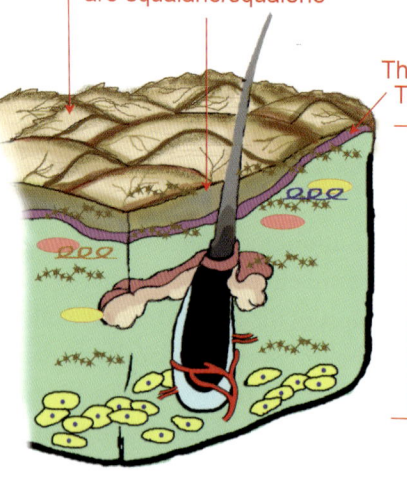

Thin acid mantle
Thin skin depth

Aged Skin

Fewer capillaries, fewer water-holding proteins, damaged collagen and elastin, thinned subcutaneous fat, diminished follicles, and fewer stem cells

: damaged proteins

© Loren Pickart PhD

Figure 1.1

What is Reverse Aging?

"Reverse aging" is a term you've probably seen before, perhaps on the back of your favorite jar of moisturizer, but what does it mean, really? Researchers will tell you that there are two types of aging: chronological aging and biological aging. To calculate our chronological age, we add up our birthdays, or the years that have passed since we were born, according to a steady clock that counts each circling of the earth around the sun as one year. But our bodies follow a different clock that measures biological age. This "biological clock" generally makes us look and feel older over time due to an inherent biological program that pushes us to age.

The good news is, under some circumstances our biological clock can go into "reverse time", when parts of the body become similar to what they were when we were younger. The body is a chemical machine and, at least in theory, most of the chemical reactions that happen with age are reversible. Physicists have claimed that some elementary particles actually go backwards in time.

A few measures you can take to slow your biological clock include regular exercise, a healthy diet, and a low level of stress. Studies show that in the United States, people live longest in small, quiet towns where little changes. Conversely, there are also conditions that can accelerate your biological clock, including psychological stress, smoking, and medical conditions such as uncontrolled diabetes. In World War I, the severe stress of trench warfare could turn a young man's hair grey in two months. The next figure and table give examples of conditions that can alter the rate of biological aging in a hypothetical person.

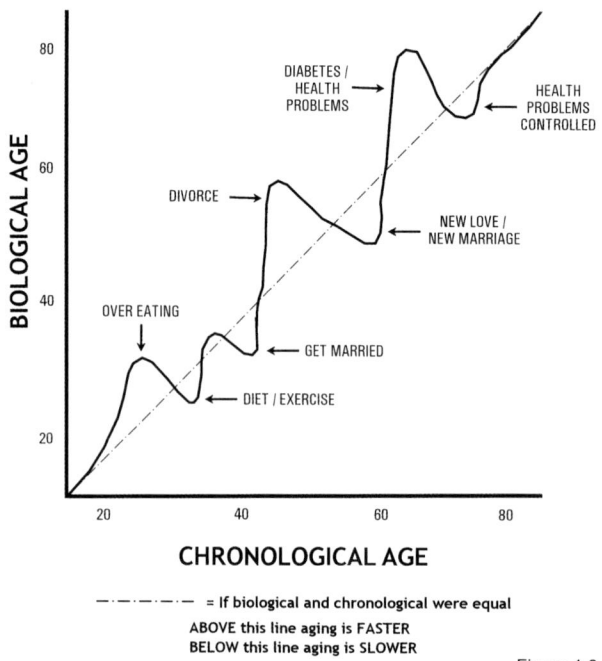

Figure 1.2

- - - = If biological and chronological were equal
ABOVE this line aging is FASTER
BELOW this line aging is SLOWER

Aging Accelerators and Aging Reversers

Increases Aging	Slows Aging
Smoking	Exercise
Fast Food	French and Italian Mediterranean Cooking
Too Few Antioxidants	Supplements of: *Vitamin E, Alpha Lipoic Acid, Coenzyme Q-10, Chelated Copper Ion*
Too Much Alcohol	Moderate Wine Consumption
Overeating	Fasting
Stressful Urban Life	Quiet Rural Life
Watching TV News	Gardening, Fishing, Reading Books
Hormone Shifts with Aging	Supplements such as DHEA
Solitary Life	Active Social Life
Stressful, Unrewarding Job	Vacations
Sun and Wind	Biological Oils, Skin Repair Products

Reverse Aging Is Within Your Grasp

The concept of aging reversal is a step beyond the anti-aging therapies that have been around for decades, such as the use of antioxidant vitamins, or a diet high in plants and low in calories. Clinical studies have proven the value of many of these anti-aging therapies in terms of maintaining a healthy lifestyle and reducing the risk of disease. The difference between anti-aging therapies and aging reversal is that the latter uses methods which actually turn back the clock on certain organs, returning them to a biological state closer to what existed at a younger age.

If the idea of reverse aging sounds too good to be true, consider the progress that has been attained by researchers in reversing certain aging effects in humans. Drugs such as Proscar reverse prostate enlargement in men. A variety of anti-lipidemic drugs can reverse the aging elevation of blood lipids that cause vascular atherosclerosis. Alpha lipoic acid, taken as a supplement, can reverse the decline in mitochondrial energy production that occurs with time.

The ideas herein are not those of traditional dermatology. They arose from studies on human aging, cell biology, and biochemical signals for regeneration, and reflect this parentage. Skin is delicate, sensitive, and fragile. At times it must be "babied" back into health. Too often, it is treated as wood or leather. Supposed "skin experts" burn it, poison it, and paint it, calling this the path to beauty. (In fact, some skin products have been marketed because they are good for the leather of horse saddles). My bias is for the biological rather than the artificial; for slow, gentle, safe treatments. In my opinion, the only worthy products are those supported by credible, independent articles in scientific journals.

As such, many of the recommendations in this book are supported by published studies from more than 40 laboratories. Cosmetic products based on my inventions have proven effective in numerous controlled, published studies for actions such as reducing fine lines, coarse wrinkles, skin lesions, excess skin, and blotchiness (mottled hyper pigmentation). They have been found to improve overall appearance, skin elasticity, firmness, clarity, thickness, damage, skin tightness, and "glow". Recommendations about my new second-generation SRCPs, such as for scar and skin-lesion reduction, are based on experiments as well as reports from clients, estheticians, and dermatologists at clinics, spas, and salons. When you see results, I hope you will drop me a line, too.

Throughout history, science has advanced through a mixture of astute observations and experimental studies. It is generally not realized that the successful theories of Newton, Einstein, and Darwin were built mainly on observation and thought. Like other scientific breakthroughs, the methods for reversing skin aging you are about to discover are accurately captured by a phrase from St. Paul: "We know in part, we prophecy in part…"

Chapter 2

Artificial and Unnatural Skin Treatments

Alien Chemicals, Junk Science, Cinderella Becomes Count Dracula

Many years ago, my mother would complain that the songbirds were no longer on our farm in Minnesota. The farm was surrounded by rolling hills and forests and had been filled with thousands of birds. But the birds started vanishing. Then, in 1962, Rachel Carson explained in *Silent Spring* that insecticides were killing bird populations. Often when I look at the list of ingredients in cosmetics, I think about the birds.

Years of raising skin cells in the laboratory, in cell culturing solutions, taught me that they are fussy and finicky about what they want. You can't just expose them to any new compound. Yet chemical companies keep spewing out alien synthetic molecules for use in cosmetics, disregarding the fact that the body has difficulty handling chemicals that have never existed inside the skin before. These new chemicals are patented and then advertised as the newest "miracle" product for the skin. They are sold not because they make the skin look better and feel healthier, but because the new molecules are patented, and thus draw a premium price.

> "The nerve inhibitors are currently numbing my cute little brain - I think they are turning me into a Stepford Wife...(or — Is this a male plot to turn us women into Stepford Wives?) but oh well, at least I'm wrinkle free. Well, I guess I better go now. I have to get back to baking cookies and trying on my new lingerie and neuropeptides."
> — Idelle Musiek

Many consumers don't realize that it is extremely difficult to improve on nature. It took 30 years of intensive research to develop effective anti-cholesterol drugs, and these still are not perfect. Most manufactured chemicals do more harm than good. For example, it isn't unusual to see a woman who, after wearing eyebrow pencil for years, has lost all her eyebrows by age 40.

Problems with alien chemicals, such as DDT and PCBs took decades to surface and still persist in the environment. This is very sad to see. For years, I have spent time every summer fishing for salmon off San Juan Island, along with the local orca pod. These friendly and inquisitive whales always come over and check out the water around my boat, *Regenerate*, to see if I have found a school of big salmon. Today, these lovely creatures are plagued by a toxic level of PCBs that threatens their very survival.

Especially dangerous are color cosmetics, such as concealers and foundations. These products are filled with a witch's brew of metallic salts, chemical dyes, optical diffusers, and alien synthetic chemicals. My advice is to use as few color cosmetics as possible. Take the money you spend on color cosmetics and spend it on jewelry, nice clothes, and attractive scents and pheromones instead. There are plenty of ways to attract attention without wreaking havoc on your skin.

Plant extracts also have many problems. If it is natural, it doesn't mean it cannot kill you. Snakes are natural, as well as poisonous plants. Plants are filled with poisons and carcinogens to avoid being eaten by hungry animals. Most exotic flowers, stems, and leaves have been shown in safety tests to be very irritating to the skin. Many carcinogens enter our body from common foods, but the gastrointestinal tract and liver are able to detoxify the dangerous ingredients in foods. The skin has no such protective system. On your skin, you should only apply plant extracts and oils that are highly domesticated, and have been used for at least a thousand years. Only a very few domesticated plants, such as aloe vera, have a positive effect on the skin.

> *"Chuck a handful of weeds in the pot and you've got herbs."*
> — Terry Pratchett

Junk Science

Cosmetic companies possess the greatest collection of Junk Science on Planet Earth. Most cosmetic companies are run by marketing people who reside in Dante's Ninth Circle (Realm of Compound Fraud) and are, consequently, beyond redemption.

Cosmetic companies announce a new miracle product about every two years. Fifty years ago, the same cosmetic companies were announcing miracle products that would remove wrinkles and stop the development of new wrinkles. What happened to the old "miracles"?

Figure 2.1

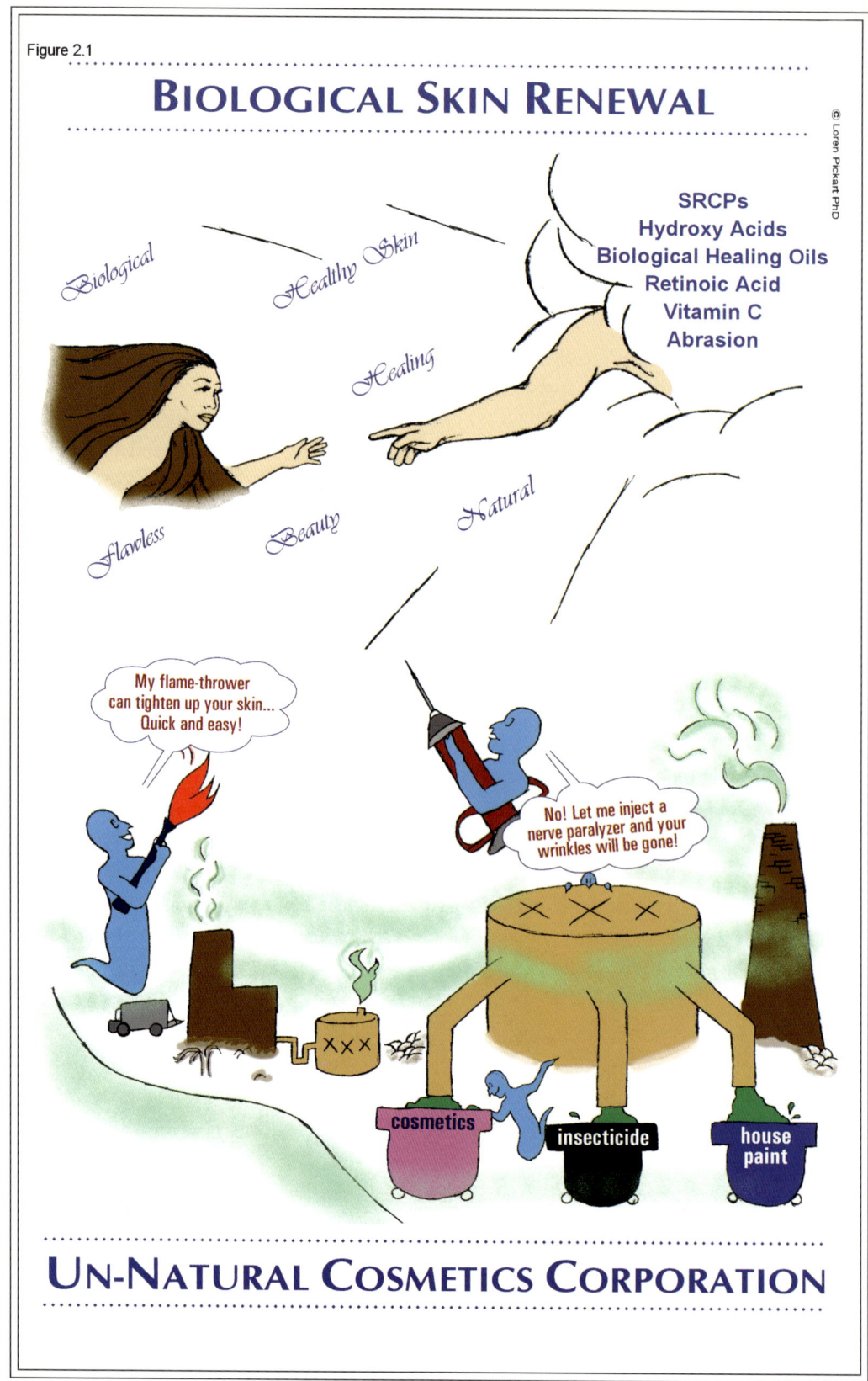

BIOLOGICAL SKIN RENEWAL

Biological *Healthy Skin*

SRCPs
Hydroxy Acids
Biological Healing Oils
Retinoic Acid
Vitamin C
Abrasion

Healing

Flawless *Beauty* *Natural*

"My flame-thrower can tighten up your skin... Quick and easy!"

"No! Let me inject a nerve paralyzer and your wrinkles will be gone!"

cosmetics insecticide house paint

UN-NATURAL COSMETICS CORPORATION

© Loren Pickart PhD

The skin-care industry tries to appear scientific. But cosmetic companies use many phrases that actually have little meaning, such as "reduces the appearance of fine wrinkles". Fine wrinkles can be reduced by any number of methods, none of which can be considered "miraculous", such as mild inflammation, bee stings, excessive sunburn, and infections.

"Clinically proven" is another badly misused phrase. Materials such as retinol, squalene, and Co-Q10 may have a positive effect on the skin when present at certain concentrations. However, even when a product contains a microscopically small and ineffective amount of one of these substances, the cosmetic companies imply that the substance's presence gives the same effect as would a larger dose. Products are manufactured for the lowest possible cost with water ("the universal extender") and cheap chemicals. Often in a "study", a product will be applied to one side of the face of a person with dry skin and nothing will be applied to the other. Under such circumstances, even simple oils would appear to have an effect on dry skin.

Extremely few of these "clinical studies" ever make it into scientific journal articles. The cosmetic industry has yet to produce even one significant discovery that has enhanced skin health. All key discoveries have been produced by private dermatologists, estheticians, academic scientists, or pharmaceutical companies. Scientists in cosmetic companies have little influence. An executive at a large cosmetic company once told me, "We pay our top scientist $180,000 per year and our top model $4 million per year. You can guess who gets listened to more".

If you were a fly on the wall at a cosmetic company, you would be shocked to discover how they make their wares. The products are ordered from generic manufacturing plants that use standard formulas. Products with similar ingredients are given different fancy names, such as Night Active Defense Cream, Anti-Gravity Skincare Lotion (this could save on airline fares if it worked), Cucumber Regenerative Tightening Gel, Natural Environmental Conditioner (how "natural" can it be with all the alien chemicals?), Stress-Reducing Lymphatic Drainage System, and so on. What links all of these products together is a lack of credible evidence that they do anything positive for the skin.

As one rather honest employee at a cosmetic company put it, "Our Anti-Wrinkle Night Cream is *philosophically* against wrinkles."

Cinderella Becomes Count Dracula

Most cosmetics are designed to make you look good at the cosmetic counter so you will buy products. Wetting agents puff up the skin so that wrinkles and lines are less noticeable. Then dyes and optical diffusers give skin a better color and "glow" and hide blemishes.

All this makes your skin look like Cinderella's at the store but like Count Dracula's in the morning. This magic trick is not akin to skin health, and sadly, often has the opposite effect of slowly degrading the skin. Many skin products sell because they feel smooth and sensuous, but this does not relate to improving skin health.

Cosmetic companies created the legend that skin "adapts" to good cosmetics and looks bad when you stop using them. But the truth is that as soon as the temporary effect is gone, you have to re-apply the cosmetics. Moisturizers designed to plump up the skin by pushing water into the skin actually damage the skin barrier by breaking the water-resistant barrier of proteins and oils of the upper skin and wetting the proteins. This weakens the skin barrier and lets in more bacteria, viruses and allergens. Also by keeping the upper skin layers wet (hydrated), the lower skin layers fail to receive the proper signals to send new cells (keratinocytes) to the surface. The result is a weakened and leaky skin.

The majority of cosmetic skin products are designed for long-term stability, that is, they can be frozen or thawed without change and have a long shelf-life, preferably years. But skin is a living tissue, and effective products need to be more like perishable foods rather than perfectly stable creams or clear solutions. Remember, expensive wine has debris at the bottom of the bottle, while cheap wine is clear.

Truth…or Fiction?

By now, you may be wondering why, if so many of the ingredients in cosmetics aren't good for us, the cosmetic industry is so successful. Unfortunately, the answer is *deception*.

Consider for a moment how many products are advertised to reduce wrinkles. Based on what you see on TV and read in magazines, it would be easy to think that every product on the market has a miraculous anti-wrinkle effect. But the cosmetic industry's main objective is to manufacture innocuous products that don't in any way irritate the skin. The cosmetic companies depend on advertising to create the illusion that their products have positive effects. Many of these products use unnatural and artificial methods to cause a sort of "skin renewal" or the appearance of skin renewal, but few are based on activating the skin's natural repair systems.

There Is No Quick Fix

While your doctor might tell you that lasers, microwaves, heating lights, and other currently popular methods of skin care induce collagen formation and, in turn, younger skin, this isn't the case. In actuality, these methods use controlled skin damage to induce new skin regeneration. Instead of causing collagen synthesis, they merely damage the skin enough so that it, hopefully, mounts a vigorous regenerative response. Sometimes they yield good results, but they can also lead to scarring and further damage. Are you willing to take the risk?

Surgical procedures, such as face lifts and implants, are followed by a long recovery period as scar lines fade and the skin adjusts to its new position. In addition, no one is sure what the future impact of such procedures will be. Remember, X-ray machines were once used to treat acne, but now, a few decades later, these patients are developing cancer from the treatment. And in the past, silicone injections were applied directly into women's faces and breasts. Later, many of these women found that the silicone slowly slid down inside their skin, necessitating surgical removal to avoid the consequence of disfigurement.

The secret to beautiful skin isn't in any of the multitudes of products or procedures you see in advertisements or hear about at the dermatology office. Rather, it is the idea that *slower is better*. Our bodies can only rebuild skin at a set pace. This is a slow process during which blemishes and damaged proteins are removed and replaced with more youthful skin.

The Skin Experts Tell Us What to Do

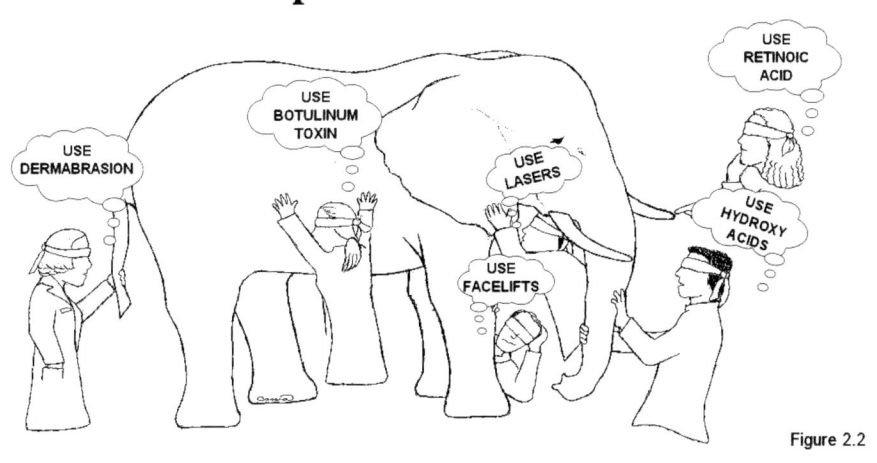

Figure 2.2

Unnatural and Artificial Methods of Skin Renewal

Method	Cell Biology and Biochemistry	Comments
Lasers: Burn off layers of skin	Gives an immediate tightening or lifting of the skin by denaturing collagen. Results depend on the skin's subsequent regenerative response. Does not directly stimulate collagen and skin tightening.	Can produce long lasting redness and scars. SRCPs are often used after procedure for better healing with less irritation. May damage vellus hair follicles and reduce stem cells for skin rebuilding.
Deep Peels: Peel away top layer of skin	Depends on skin's subsequent regenerative response. Does not directly stimulate collagen and skin tightening.	Can produce long lasting redness and scars. SRCPs are often used after procedure for better healing with less irritation.
Strong Dermabrasion: Removes top layer of skin	Depends on skin's subsequent regenerative response. Does not directly stimulate collagen and skin tightening.	Can produce long lasting redness and scars. SRCPs are often used after procedure for better healing with less irritation.
Microwaves and Infra-red Machines	Contracts collagen like bacon in a pan.	Put some bacon in a bowl and turn on your kitchen microwave.
Skin Fillers: Injectable	Injection of large molecules like modified bovine collagen, "non-animal" derived hyaluronic acid (from bacteria) and poly-lactic acid (from bacteria).	Rapid action on filling defects but must be repeated about every six months. May produce bumpy skin and allergies. Hyaluronic acid speeds the spread of many cancers.
Skin Fillers: Topical	Creams with peptides: aminopeptides, pentapeptides, etc., that act like Transforming Growth Factor beta 1, which causes scar formation, causes normal cells to grow like cancer cells, and may speed the spread of breast cancer.	Increases skin proteins but does not remove old proteins. Can produce hard spots and bumps in skin. Products like these were tested for wound healing but produced heavy scarring.
Nerve Paralyzers: Injectable	Injection of botulinum toxin.	Must be repeated every six months. End with inelastic skin and paralyzed muscles. Can produce new wrinkles at edges in injected area. Gets into brain.
Nerve Paralyzers: Topical	Creams with short action nerve blockers.	Anti-wrinkle effect lasts about 8 hours. Safety questions about continuous use of nerve paralyzers.
Surgical Methods	Face lifts, skin tightening.	Works well with extensive loose skin. Painful and costly.
Artificial Implants	Implants.	Permanent improvement in skin contour. Implants may fail.
Color Cosmetics	Quick and cheap. Makes skin look good at cosmetic counter in stores.	The dyes and colored metal salts and wetting (hydrating) agents produce skin damage over time.
Moisturizers that wet (hydrate) skin's outer proteins	Quickly makes the skin look better.	Damages the skin's protective layer with time, allowing the entry of wart-causing viruses and pathological bacteria.
Cosmetic Skin Renewal and Regenerating Products	Ask for published, independent studies on these products in science journals before buying.	The cosmetic companies have had new "miracle skin products" for over 50 years. If they told the truth in the past, why would anyone have wrinkles today?

Chapter 3

Remodeling - The Key To Youthful Skin

Why Do Children Have Such Beautiful Skin?

Have you ever heard someone describe something as being "soft as a baby's bottom"? People use this expression for a reason. Children have the most beautiful skin: soft, firm, elastic, and blemish-free. When a child's skin is damaged, the scars usually fade within a week or two.

The reason children have such gorgeous skin is a process called skin remodeling. It is the same process that removes scars and damaged skin during adult wound repair. Damaged skin is repaired and replaced with new, blemish-free skin. In children, this process functions efficiently and skin damage, blemishes, and imperfections are rapidly removed. But, to our disadvantage, in adults skin remodeling slows drastically.

As we age, a number of changes occur to our skin. These include:

1. A reduced rate of cell replacement, producing a thinner, more fragile skin.
   Skin is replaced every three weeks at age 20 but only every nine weeks by age 70.

2. A decreased effectiveness of the protective antioxidant systems. These can drop by 80 percent between ages 15 and 60.

3. An accumulation of damaged proteins. This damage can be the result of scars, sun damage, oxidative damage, or the cross-linking of skin proteins by sugars.

4. A reduced rate of oil production. This means less acne, but dryer skin. The drop in oil production begins around age 25 and becomes more dramatic after age 45.

5. A decreased production of water-holding proteins and an increased breakdown of collagen and elastin. Wrinkle formation and loss of elasticity begins around age 25. The problem becomes progressively more serious with passing years.

6. A reduction in the size and efficiency of the vellus hair follicles. This fine, color-less hair covers most of the body surface, supplying new stem cells for skin repair.

Battling these changes by avoiding damage to the skin is not an adequate approach. While taking steps to protect your skin from ultraviolet light, allergens, detergents, damaging soaps, irritants, acne scars, airborne pollutants, chemical sun-screens, and so on will reduce some types of skin damage, this is only one piece of a much larger puzzle. You can hide from the sun until you evolve into a mole, but this will not keep your skin young.

When children are sunburned or have skin injuries that cause scars, they do not develop wrinkled and blemished skin because the damage is quickly removed. So it makes sense that the secret to youthful skin lies in enhancing the skin remodeling process in adults.

THE LAYERS OF OUR SKIN

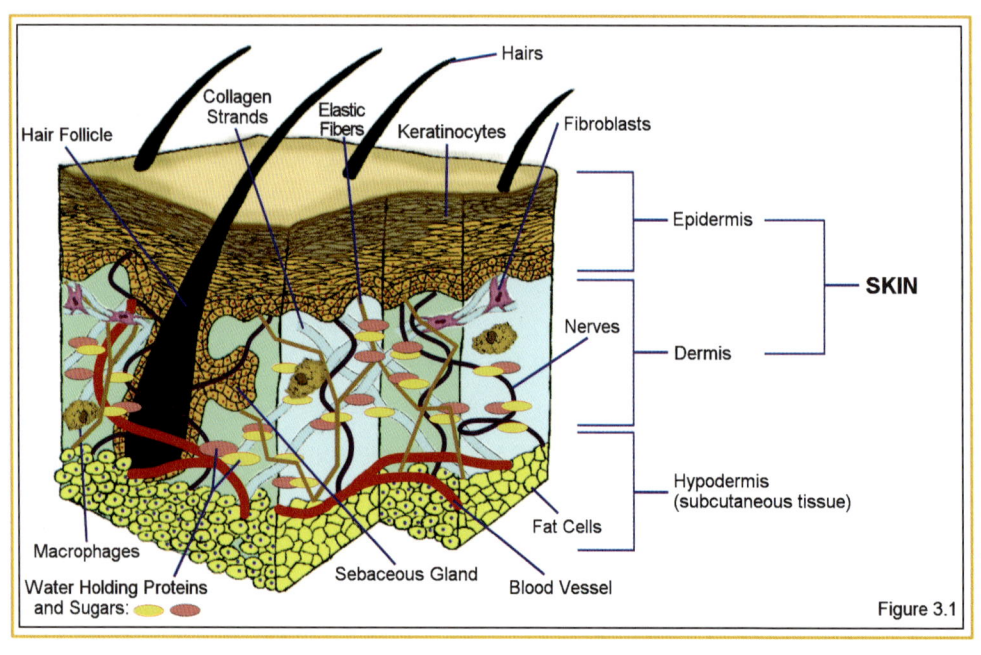

Figure 3.1

SKIN	Effect of Aging	Effect of Skin Remodeling
	Thinner, more fragile skin	Thickened skin – dermis and epidermis
	Less elastic skin	Rebuilt new collagen and elastin
	Less subcutaneous fat "baby fat"	Increased subcutaneous fat
	More skin lesions, imperfections, blotchiness	Activate scar removal system that removes lesions and scars
	Poor blood capillary networks	Rebuilt capillary networks for better tissue nutrition
	Flabby, less firm skin	Increased synthesis of water-holding proteins
HAIR	Less hair growth	Increased hair growth
	Smaller hair follicle size	Increased follicle size
	Thinner hair shafts	Thicker hair shafts
	More breakage of hair shafts and split ends	Thicker, more break resistant hair shafts

The Holy Grail of Skin Care

Cosmetic products that effectively produce skin remodeling are the Holy Grail of skin care. Although there are many skin remodeling techniques, most have drawbacks. Retinoic acid (Retin-A) slowly remodels skin, but at the price of chronic irritation and redness. Certain peptides, melatonin, and topical vitamin C increase collagen, but the skin also needs replacement of elastin and water-holding proteoglycans, and its microcirculation must be rebuilt. A class of peptides that function like TGF-ß-1, the scar-forming growth factor, increase the skin's extracellular matrix proteins and was extensively tested in the 1990's for wound healing, but produced unacceptable skin thickening and scarring because they do not adequately remove older pre-existing proteins. Lasers, chemical peels, and dermabrasion work well only if there is a vigorous post-therapy regenerative response from the damaged skin.

The Skin's Natural Renewal Systems and Protectants

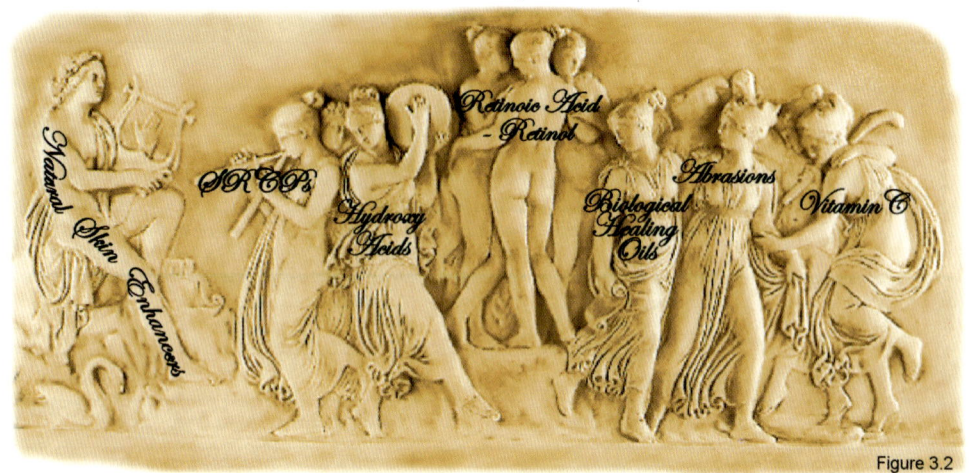

Figure 3.2

Maximizing the Skin's Natural Renewal Systems

Research indicates that skin health and remodeling depends on only a relatively few number of biological compounds. Our skin has used a very small set of molecules and renewal effectors for at least 230 million years. Birds and mammals heal similarly. Their ancestors diverged at this time. The skin does not change its biochemistry every two years for new advertising campaigns from cosmetic companies that promise dramatic results for aging women and men, but then use 25-year-old models in their ads because the products really do nothing.

Our skin has powerful natural systems that renew themselves, remove blemishes and scars, and tighten the skin. In skin remodeling, the goal is to use these natural activators as much as possible. There are several ingredients and methods that maximize the skin's natural renewal systems. These ingredients and methods are described in the following chart and the remainder of this chapter.

Natural Activators	Cell Biology and Biochemistry	Comments
Skin Remodeling Copper-Peptides (SRCPs) Used in human body - Exist in tissues, plasma and saliva	1. Anti-inflammatory — Blocks Interleukin-1, TGF-beta-1, and release of oxidizing iron. Detoxifies free radicals. 2. Activates removal of damaged proteins, scars, and blemishes. 3. Helps synthesis of new collagen, elastin, and water-holding molecules for firmer, more elastic skin. 4. Helps rebuild microcirculation for better skin nutrition and youthful "glow". 5. Helps tighten collagen strands and tightens loose skin. 6. Repairs skin barrier to be more protective against viruses and bacteria, and lose less moisture. 7. May increase production of stem cells for the skin. 8. Increases proliferation of fibroblasts and keratinocytes.	Very safe
Exfoliating Hydroxy Acids	Normally on and in skin. Lactic acid and salicylic acid are normally in the skin.	Irritating if used excessively.
Biological Skin Oils	Emu oil is similar to human skin oils. Squalane is normally in the skin.	Emu oil and squalane have proven healing effects.
Retinoic Acid	Normally in skin. Proven to remodel skin but may act by irritation and exfoliation. Role in skin appears to help differentiate stem cells into skin cells.	Often used with SRCPs for better effects with less irritation.
Vitamin C	Normally in skin. Acts with copper(II) to tighten collagen strands.	Best if taken as supplement of 500 mg to 1 gram daily.
Mild Abrasion	Like cleansing or rubbing. Animals do this to speed skin renewal.	Very safe.

About Your Skin's Natural Renewal Activators

1. Magic Molecules: Skin Remodeling Copper Peptides (SRCPs)

SRCPs are essential to skin and tissue remodeling. They are exceptionally safe and gentle. There is nothing else like them in the human body. It is important to note that not all copper peptides are SRCPs. I have analyzed and tested some other types of copper peptides and found little or no activity. And some copper peptides can even be toxic to the skin.

As I described in Chapter 1, SRCPs help trigger the skin's natural mechanism of renewal and restore the skin to a biologically younger and healthier condition. We have learned a lot about SRCPs in the past two decades. The first SRCP that I discovered and used for skin remodeling was a small peptide-copper complex, present in human blood, saliva, and urine. This blue colored molecule, technically called GHK-Cu (glycyl-l-histidyl-l-lysine:copper(II)), reversed certain effects of aging in human and animal experiments. In 1984, I and a few of my colleagues started a company, Procyte (Latin "for-the cell"), to develop GHK-Cu into useful products. It is now used in cosmetic and hair-care products and after clinical skin-renewal procedures such as chemical peels, laser resurfacing, and dermabrasion to improve post-treatment skin recovery.

The GHK-Cu Breakthrough

The wound healing and anti-inflammatory actions of GHK-Cu were the first actions I investigated. But by 1989, I discovered, using a pilot study of 20 women, that skin creams containing GHK-Cu increased the thickness of the dermis and epidermis, increased elasticity, reduced wrinkles, and resulted in the removal of imperfections, such as blotchiness and sun damage, while producing a significant increase in subcutaneous fat cells. This new information was used to obtain a patent on the cosmetic uses of GHK-Cu.

Unfortunately, these observations languished for another 10 years. There was a general disbelief among skin-care researchers that a single biochemical compound could both heal wounds and improve the cosmetic quality of intact skin. Since then, numerous studies have established GHK-Cu's wound-healing properties. Between 2002 and 2005, nine placebo-controlled studies by leading dermatologists were published, confirming GHK-Cu's reversal of aging actions on human skin. At long last, an increasing number of researchers are realizing that one SRCP can both heal broken and damaged skin and improve the quality of intact undamaged skin. (See references in Chapter 16).

Based on GHK-Cu, clinical studies have found that SRCPs have the following cosmetic actions on the skin:
- Calming irritated and reddened skin
- Tightening loose skin and improving elasticity
- Tightening the protective skin barrier proteins
- Improving skin firmness
- Reducing fine lines
- Reducing the depth of deep wrinkles
- Improving skin clarity and "glow"
- Reducing spots, photodamage, and hyperpigmentation
- Smoothing rough skin
- Improving overall appearance

Cosmetic products that contain GHK-Cu include lines such as Visibly Firm® by Neutrogena and Neova® by Procyte.

Second-Generation SRCPs

Although products containing GHK-Cu performed well in many tests, these products failed FDA clinical trials on difficult-to-heal human wounds (as have many other approaches). GHK-Cu's actions are limited by fragility and a tendency toward breakdown, as well as a lack of adhesion to the skin's surface.

Therefore, in 1994, I started Skin Biology to develop improved second-generation SRCPs with enhanced potency, breakdown resistance, and high adherence to the skin. I isolated peptide fragments from soy protein digests that possessed the desired qualities when chelated to copper(II). Such peptides are very non-allergic and have a long history of safe use in cosmetic products.

In my tests, the second-generation of SRCPs has proven to be even more effective than the first. In veterinary studies, creams made from the new SRCPs produced rapid and scar-free healing in dogs after spaying operations and in young horses after leg-straightening operations. At the University of California, San Francisco, Howard Maibach and colleagues tested these new copper peptides in four small, placebo-controlled human studies. They found that creams made from the complexes produced significantly faster healing and reduced redness and inflammation after mild skin injuries.

Our work on the new SRCPs had an unexpected result. Somewhat accidentally, women and men began using them for cosmetic purposes and reported improved skin condition and hair vitality. When the breakdown-resistant SRCPs were used with hydroxy acids, many types of blemishes and scars were slowly removed from the skin. This discovery was followed by many reports from clients of wrinkle reduction, skin tightening, and improved hair growth and condition.

SRCPs and Wound Healing

SRCPs and their relationship to skin remodeling is best understood within the context of wound healing. Cosmetic remodeling of uninjured skin appears to be similar to remodeling after wounding. Numerous studies have demonstrated that SRCPs accelerate the healing of wounds and damaged skin and also cause strong remodeling of intact, undamaged skin. (For more details see Chapter 16).

The human body uses the same biochemical mechanisms for closely related purposes. Many dermatological techniques used for skin remodeling (such as lasers, dermabrasion, and chemical peels) actually induce a mild wounding to trigger the remodeling process.

WOUND HEALING

Figure 3.4

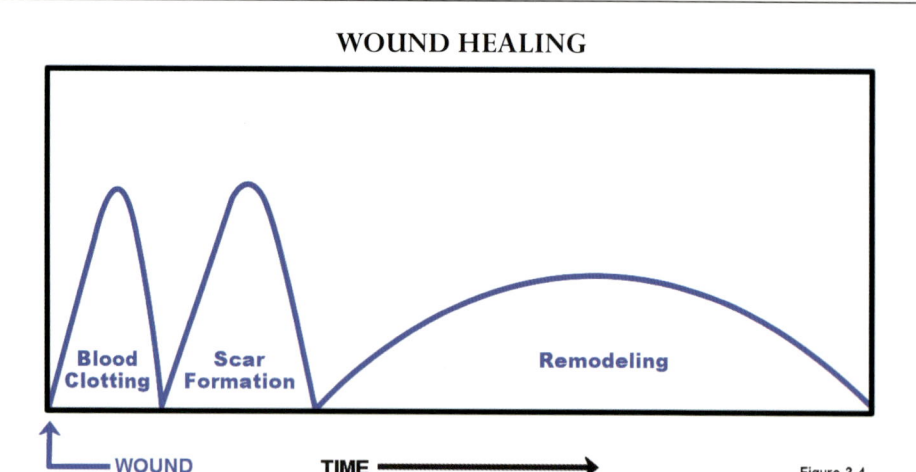

- Blood Clotting
- Scar Formation
- Remodeling
- WOUND
- TIME

SRCPs: • Stimulating Wound Healing
• Activating Remodeling of Intact Skin

(Not all copper-peptides and copper complexes are SRCPs, some used in cosmetics actually inhibit skin repair)

Excitingly, research shows that this same mechanism can be used to reduce wrinkles.

Example of Reversing Skin Aging by Skin Remodeling

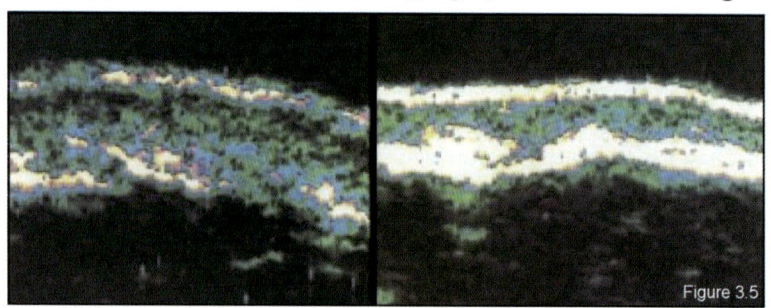

Figure 3.5

SRCPs Really Work!

The application of SRCP complexes to the skin's surface creates an environment that helps the skin tighten its barrier and increase its collagen production and elastin density. The photo above on the left is an ultrasound scan of the skin of a woman age 59. On the right is a photo showing the same woman after one month of treatment with a cream containing SRCPs. The white-yellow colored areas are the ultrasonic reflection from skin areas that are more dense because of closer cellular binding and increased amounts of collagen and elastin. This is the opposite effect of the usual thinning and loosening of skin produced by aging.

2. Exfoliating Hydroxy Acids (EHAs)

Exfoliating hydroxy acids are often used to increase SRCP effects and to loosen older skin and scar tissue. The most natural EHAs are lactic acid and salicylic acid. Both exist naturally in the skin and on the skin's surface and act to loosen the chemical links between older skin cells and allow for their removal. This prompts the skin cells to move to the surface and speeds up skin renewal.

The practice of using EHAs is very old. In the ancient book *Beautification*, Cleopatra described the use of fruit acids, sour wine, and sour milk (all of which contain EHAs) to renew and beautify the skin. The book was a "best-seller" for 200 years. Today, we use pure forms of such exfoliating skin acids, the alpha hydroxy acids (AHAs) and the beta hydroxy acids (BHAs) to speed up skin turnover, remove skin lesions, and restore the skin's firmness, elasticity, and internal moisture-holding properties.

Exfoliating Hydroxy Acids: EHA

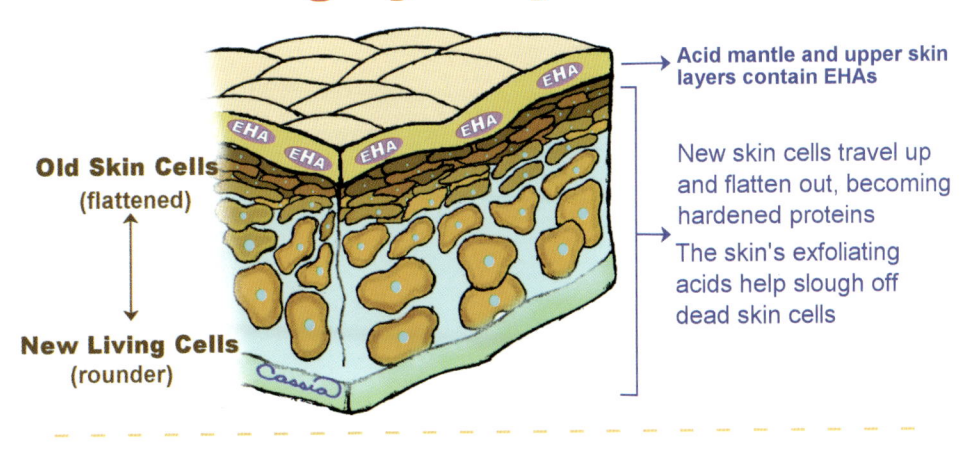

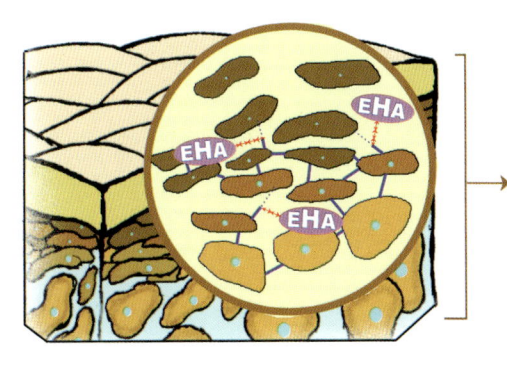

Old Skin Cells (flattened)
New Living Cells (rounder)

- Acid mantle and upper skin layers contain EHAs
- New skin cells travel up and flatten out, becoming hardened proteins
- The skin's exfoliating acids help slough off dead skin cells

Exfoliating Hydroxy Acids: Break intercellular links and old cells slough off

As EHA removes old cells, younger cells move to skin's surface

© Loren Pickart PhD

Figure 3.6

3. Biological Healing Oils (BHOs)

Biological Healing Oils exist naturally in the skin and on the skin's surface. The oils waterproof the skin. They also help repair the skin barrier by acting as a glue that binds the outer skin proteins together and keeps them relatively dry so that they are hard and protective. It has been compared to thinking of the proteins as bricks in a wall and the BHOs as the concrete holding them together. BHOs are excellent topical moisturizers that act by blocking excessive water loss from the skin. Unfortunately, these naturally occurring oils lessen as we age.

BHOs can be used to modulate SRCP uptake by the skin. For example, an SRCP product (such as Skin Biology's CP Serum) can be applied, and then after the serum dries a little, followed with a BHO, which pushes more SRCPs into the skin or hair follicle. To reduce SRCP effects on irritated skin, the BHO can be applied before the SRCP. In this manner, the BHO will reduce the uptake of the SRCPs and produce a milder effect.

Emu oil (such as Skin Biology's Emu Oil-S) is similar to the BHOs generated by human skin. This oil has been used by Australian native peoples for thousands of years for moisturizing and healing.

True Skin Moisturization
A long term enhancement of skin health, suppleness, and softness

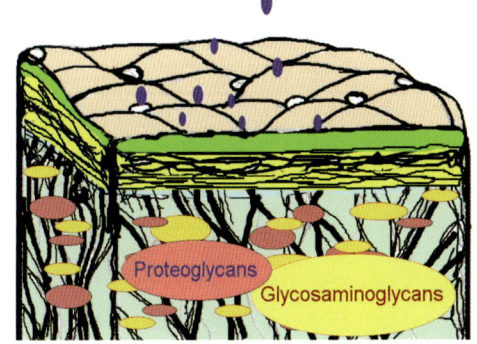

Evaporating H_2O ← Light water loss through skin

Skin is covered with thick acid mantle of oils, acids, and water.

Skin barrier is highly protective due to proteins glued together by lipids.

Many water-holding Glycosaminoglycans and Proteoglycans

False Cosmetic Moisturization
Quickly makes skin attractive at cosmetic sales counter, but slowly damages the skin inhibiting normal skin renewal and producing a daily moisturizer need somewhat like a drug addiction

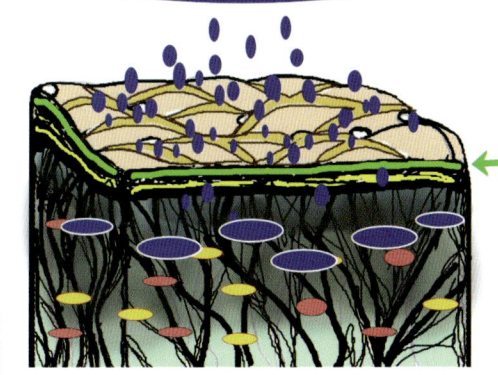

Evaporating H_2O ← If you stop using these products, then a very high water loss through the skin results

Detergents thin acid mantle

Detergents remove acid mantle and disrupt the skin barrier's wall of proteins and lipids. The proteins become weak and wet (hydrated) by water pushed into the skin.

Few water-holding Glycosaminoglycans and Proteoglycans

The wetness of the upper skin layers stops the signals to the lower layers to produce more skin cells to move to the surface and reduces the production of water holding molecules in the skin.

Figure 3.7

4. Retinoic Acid and Retinol

Retinoic acid is used for skin remodeling in drug products such as Retin-A and Renova. Retinol is vitamin A and is also used in many skin products. There is much confusion over these two compounds, which is deliberately fostered by cosmetic companies. The following chart highlights the differences between the two.

	Retinoic Acid	**Retinol**
Chemical name	Retinoic acid	Retinyl alcohol
Common name	Vitamin A acid	Vitamin A
Prescription Drugs	Retin-A	Not a drug
Effect on skin oil	Reduces skin oil	Increases skin oil
Effect on wrinkles	Strong wrinkle reduction	Mild effect on reduction of fine lines

The skin's natural retinoic acid appears to cause the skin's stem cells to differentiate into adult cells such as fibroblasts and keratinocytes. While retinoic acid is used for skin remodeling, this effect may be due to its irritating actions, which speed cell turnover.

Many people use SRCPs and retinoic acid products together and report better results with less irritation. Creams with retinol (usually a retinol derivative, such as retinyl palmitate) are sold for wrinkle reduction but have only very modest effects. Retinol has been used in skin creams for more than 60 years, yet consumers still get wrinkles.

I have found that, in general, products with a low level of retinol seem to increase skin oils and work very well for people over age 40 with drier skin. But retinol can cause increased acne in persons between ages 18 and 30. Paradoxically, clients between ages 25 and 40 often report that retinol creams help with chronic cystic acne. When using retinol cream, it is best to start slowly and work up to a higher dose.

5. Vitamin C (Ascorbic Acid)

Our tissue cells use vitamin C and a copper enzyme called lysyl oxidase to cross-link and tighten collagen. This activity depends on your system having adequate amounts of both copper(II) and vitamin C. It is best to put the copper products on the skin and raise your vitamin C levels with oral supplements of 0.5 to 1 gram daily since increased vitamin C is easily tolerated by the body. We need about 20 milligrams of vitamin C daily to stay alive, but studies of the natural diets of other primates suggests that 5 grams per day would be a better dosage for humans.

6. Mild Abrasion

Various forms of skin abrasion, a mild rubbing or scrubbing of the skin, remove older skin and blemishes and help the skin rebuild. Animals often will rub against a tree or fence post to help heal areas of the skin that are damaged. Abrasion is natural, and the skin is well built to respond to abrasive rubbing and slight damage by launching a strong regenerative skin-repair response. Methods such as microdermabrasion, a very mild abrasion of the skin's upper surface, have proven very effective.

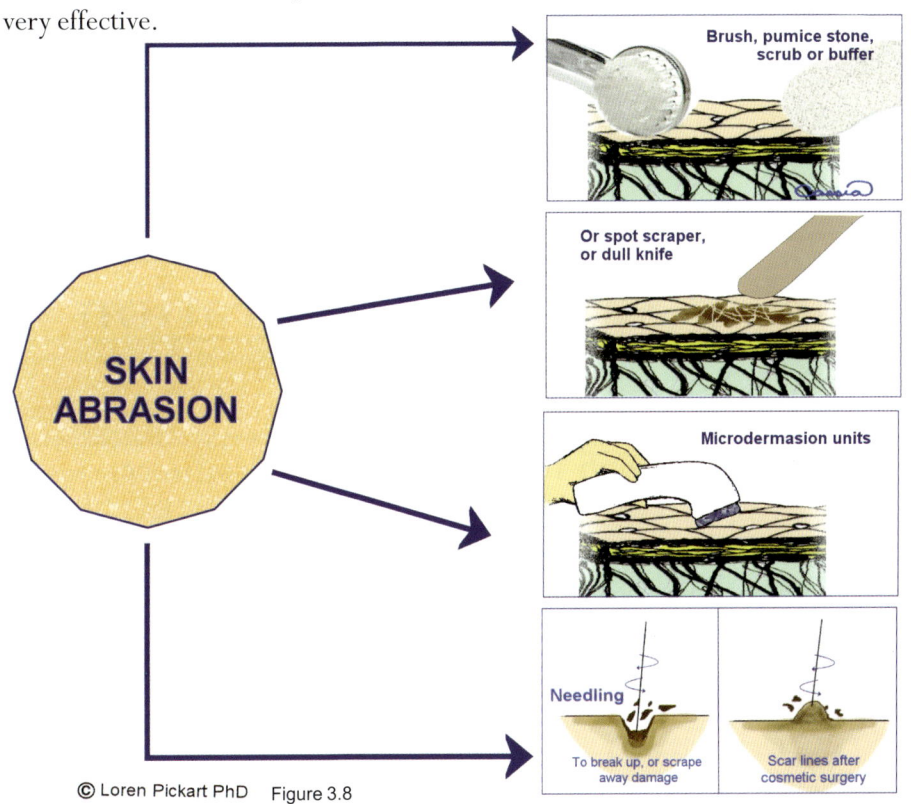

© Loren Pickart PhD   Figure 3.8

A Note on Protective Antioxidants and Avoiding Artificial Antioxidants

Protective antioxidants also have their role in skin products. But stick to those normally used in the human body such as the vitamin E family, the tocotrienol family, lutein, lycopene, CoQ-10 and alpha-lipoic acid. Our body has learned what is needed over several hundred million years. Exotic antioxidants, that the body did not choose to use, are a risk. Avoid artificial antioxidants that are advertised as more potent than the body's natural antioxidants. While free radicals can damage skin and other tissues, they are needed in many key reactions within the body. For example, free radicals are needed by the immune cells to kill bacteria, viruses, and cancer cells and by the mitochondria to produce energy. Some artificial antioxidants are so powerful that they cause tissue damage by shutting down key reactions and some have produced cancer.

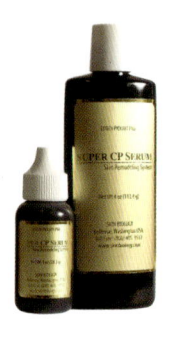

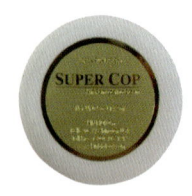

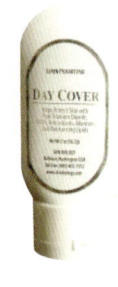

Chapter 4

Using Second-Generation SRCPs

My Approach to Making Skin Products

Y ou now know that the cosmetic industry doesn't have your best interests at heart and that second-generation SRCPs are the key to younger-looking, healthier skin. In this chapter, you will discover the most effective methods for natural skin renewal and the recommended Skin Biology products for turning back the clock on your skin.

One note: I give only general recommendations for the use of Skin Biology products because, like everything in life, you have to experiment to discover what works best for your individual skin. That's because each of us is unique. You could have an identical twin with the same DNA and yet react differently to the same products because of differences in diet, stress level, the condition of your skin, and your skin's previous exposure to allergens. My advice is to keep experimenting until you find the combination of products that works best for you.

Figure 4.1

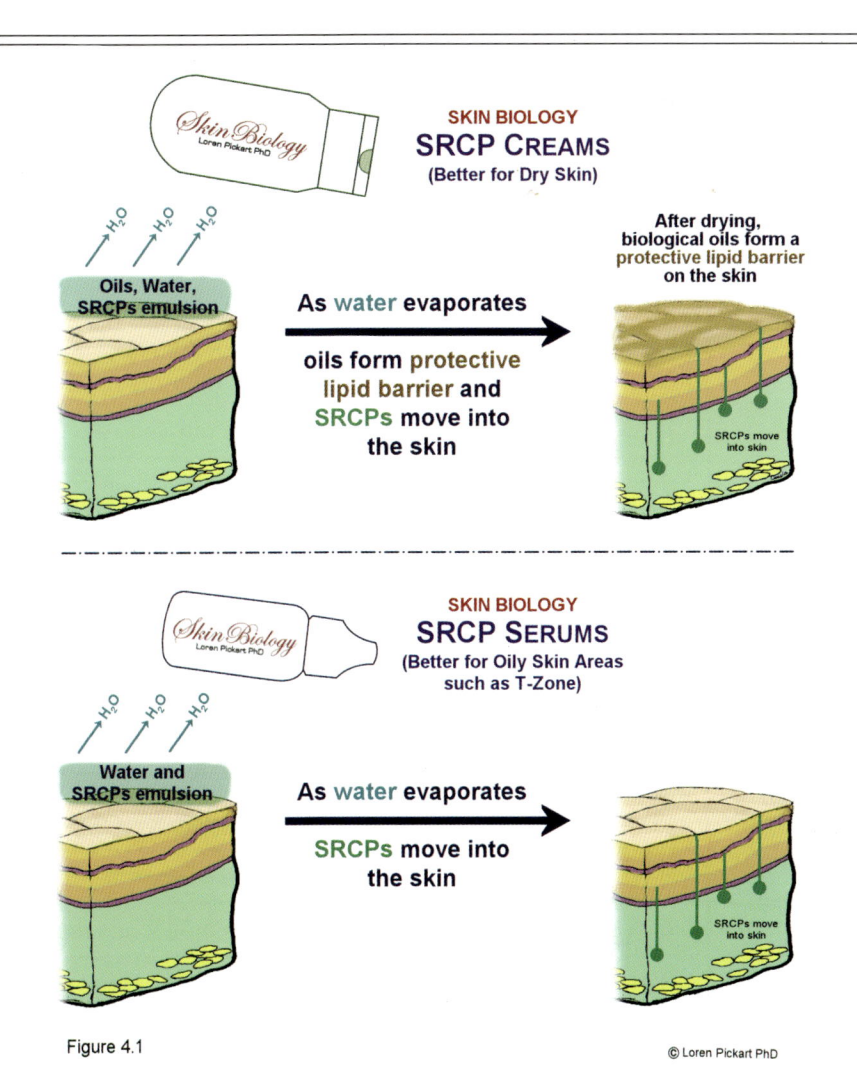

Damaged Skin Must Be Babied Back To Health

The Golden Rule of SRCPs is to start lightly and increase gradually. As your skin barrier is repaired and rebuilt, your skin will become more protective and fewer materials, including SRCPs, will be able to penetrate it.

The area around the eyes is especially delicate. This skin is very thin, and for many people has been severely damaged over the years by exposure to harsh color cosmetics and make-up removers. As your skin adjusts to the application of SRCPs, you can transition to stronger products if your skin needs a more intensive rebuilding.

The following chart describes the relative strength of SRCPs in Skin Biology products and their various uses. Many people start with CP Serum, and then as their skin becomes stronger, progress on to Super CP Serum, and finally on to Super Cop.

Relative Strength of SRCPs in Skin Biology Products

Strength	Products	Use
Very Mild	CP Night Eyes Premier	For under eye area use
Mild	CP Night Eyes	For under eye area use
Mild	Protect & Restore Body Lotion	For body skin
Mild	Protect & Restore Day Cover	Fortified with UV reflector and anti-oxidants
Moderate	CP Serum	Good on oily skin
Moderate	Protect & Restore - Classic	Facial cream for under age 35
Moderate	Protect & Restore - with Retinol	Facial cream for dry skin over age 35
Strong	TriReduction Basic	Better on oily skin
Strong	TriReduction with Retinol	Better on dry skin
Strong	Protect & Restore BND Cream	Breasts, Nipples, Décolletage area (also good on neck area)
Strong	BioHeal	Good on sensitive or irritated skin
Strong	Super CP Serum	Good on acne prone skin
Very Strong	Super Cop Cream	Strong remodeling system
Very Strong	Super Cop 2X - Extra Strength	Strongest remodeling system
Strong	Folligen Cream	Good for hairline and eyebrows
Strong	Folligen Lotion	Good for irritated scalp
Strong	Folligen Spray	Use on un-irritated scalp

It is best to start with a milder product and slowly progress to a stronger product if needed.

The Signs of SRCPs at Work

As your skin adjusts to the SRCPs (particularly when they are combined with hydroxy acids), there may be a brief period of skin loosening of about two weeks before the skin tightens. Damaged skin can be somewhat like hard scar tissue, and its toughness holds everything in place. As the damaged skin is removed, your skin may briefly loosen before it is pulled tight by the production of new collagen and elastin. Skin fibroblasts first produce collagen and elastin, and then the fibroblasts slowly pull the protein strands together and tighten the skin.

You might also notice that deeply buried scar tissue becomes exposed. Old scar tissue is often covered over with normal skin; for example, cystic acne can form hard scars under the skin, which are later covered by superficial skin cells. As the skin is exfoliated, this old, buried scar tissue can become visible. Using SRCPs and hydroxy acids on the problem areas will help remove this buried damage.

If the skin becomes loose, or puffy, effectively rest the skin from SRCPs for a time by using only a biological oil such as Emu Oil-S or Squalane. Or a light DMAE (dimethylaminoethanol) serum can be used. The DMAE helps to tighten the area and usually is based in a biological oil as well, such as 5% DMAE in squalane. Then slowly return to the use of the SRCPs. Periodically resting the skin in this manner has worked well for many people going through this transition period of skin renewal.

Tips for Natural Skin Renewal

The following products and methods will help optimize your results.

If you have sensitive skin and want to decrease the activity of SRCPs, start by applying a biological healing oil. When a BHO, such as Emu Oil-S (supplemented with the skin's natural antioxidants) or Squalane, is used before SRCPs, the effect is reduced because the oils penetrate the skin and form an oil barrier that slows the SRCP uptake into your skin. This method is often used for irritated or very sensitive skin, such as after laser burns or deep peels.

To increase the activity of SRCPS, for example, if you have been using Skin Biology products for a while, follow the product application with a biological healing oil. When a BHO, such as Emu Oil-S or Squalane, is used after SRCPs, the effect is increased because the oil pushes more SRCPs into the skin. This method is often used around the eyes. Emu Oil-S and Squalane are also helpful in removing make-up and are much better for your skin than the make-up removers manufactured by cosmetic companies.

Using exfoliating hydroxy acids can help increase rebuilding and loosen older skin and scar tissue. Hydroxy acids exist naturally on the skin's surface. Lactic acid and salicylic acids are the most natural. Normally one product is used in the morning and the other at night. Stronger hydroxy acids work faster, but overuse can be irritating. Some people use SRCPs one day and hydroxy acids on alternate days. Exfol Serum contains salicylic acid plus antioxidants and is best for oily skin areas. Exfol Cream also has salicylic acid plus protective lipids, such as squalane and octyl-palmitate.

Abrasion can help remove lesions. Skin is normally subject to various types of abrasion and mild damage that stimulate removal of scars and older skin. Abrasive methods available at the doctor's office include dermabrasion, which helps remove elevated and flat scars and lesions; and needling (subcision), which removes and loosens scar tissue in depressed scars and pitted acne. At-home abrasion methods include microdermasion units, files, and pumice stones.

Using Biological Healing Oils to Modulate SRCPs

Figure 1: Milder Effect
Apply Oil First
Apply SRCPs on Top

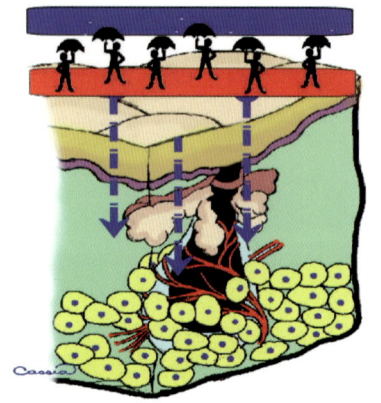

Blue: SRCPs
Red: BHOs

When first starting SRCPs for skin renewal:
Slow down SRCP penetration by applying
biological healing oils lightly before SRCPs

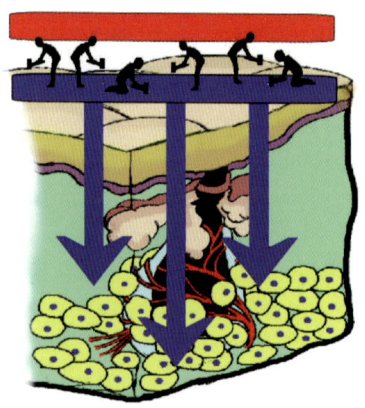

Figure 2: Stronger Effect
Apply SRCPs First
Apply Oil on Top

After a period of time for enhanced results:
Apply biological healing oils after applying
SRCPs to skin to increase SRCP uptake

© Loren Pickart PhD

Figure 4.2

My approach to making skin products:

1. All products are designed to help improve skin health. Many cosmetic products slowly degrade skin health. Our approach emphasizes the skin's natural activators of renewal and remodeling: SRCPs, hydroxy acids, natural biological oils that are in the skin, types of skin abrasion, retinoic acid, and vitamin C (this is best taken internally). What actually triggers the skin's renewal responses is a rather narrow list.

2. Our basic SRCP products have been tested by independent laboratories and been classified as non-irritants, non-allergens, non-carcinogenic, and non-poisonous. Skin Biology water/oil creams have no detergents and are always close to breaking up into a water phase and oil phase. They do not open and damage the skin barrier. Four published studies found they increase the skin barrier strength.

3. The selection of ingredients and formulations that improve skin health are based on published studies in reputable science journals by ourselves and others.

4. We select ingredients from the FDA's GRAS (Generally Recognized As Safe) list of food ingredients and cosmetic ingredients with a long history of product safety. The FDA states that safety information exists on only 11 percent of the 10,500 cosmetic ingredients cataloged by the FDA.

5. FDA requirements call for the use of formulations that resist bacterial growth. We use preservatives with long records of safety in cosmetic products.

6. We avoid the following:

6.1 Formulations and moisturizers that are designed to push water into the skin, wet the outer skin proteins, and "puff up" the skin to make wrinkles and creases less obvious. The problem is that as such products loosen and wet the skin, they damage the skin barrier and permit easier access by bacteria, viruses, and allergens. The chronic wetness also inhibits the signals that tell the skin to send more keratinocytes to the surface.

6.2 "New chemical entities", that is, synthetic molecules that the human body has never been previously exposed to in our history. It requires decades to determine the safety of such molecules, such as in the case of PCBs and DDT.

6.3 Plant extracts, with the exception of a few ingredients such as aloe vera that have exceptionally good records of non-allergic actions on skin. Plant extracts are alien to human skin and, in time, may cause rashes and allergic reactions.

6.4 Types of collagen-inducing peptides that act like Transforming Factor Beta-1, a protein named because it caused normal cells to grow like cancer cells. Concerns have been raised that such types of molecules may speed the spread of cancers and play a role in kidney failure.

6.5 Hyaluronic acid (hyaluronan) because it plays a critical role in the spread of cancer cells.

6.6 Ingredients used as nerve inhibitors to relax muscles to reduce wrinkles. Long term cosmetic use of such ingredients may inhibit nerve function in the brain and other areas of the body.

6.7 Dyes and coloring agents.

6.8 Chemical sunscreen oils. (See Chapter 14).

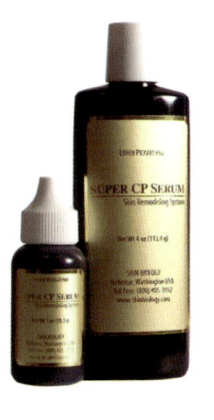

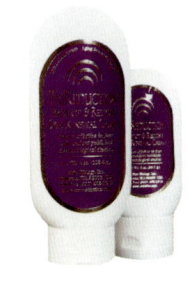

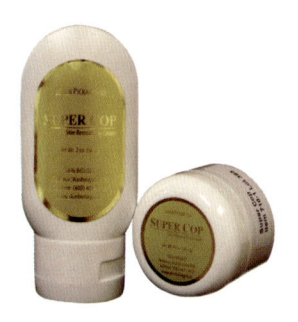

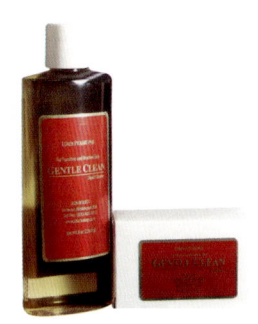

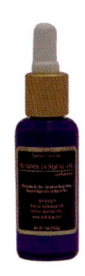

Chapter 5

Why Wrinkles Develop and How to Remove Them

Your Body's Natural Wrinkle Removal System

Most people believe wrinkles to be an unfortunate sign of aging that, as the years pass, we all must deal with. With SRCPs, however, this doesn't have to be the case. Remember, SRCPs were discovered in the field of wound healing. This background makes them very effective in dealing with the type of skin repair required to naturally decrease the appearance of wrinkles.

To understand how SRCPs work, it helps to know how a wrinkle develops. There are several types of wrinkles (static, dynamic, and mimic wrinkles); and the loss of skin moisture also produces fine lines. But all these wrinkles and lines develop when the skin's elasticity, firmness, and thickness decrease. When you stroke a child's skin, you will notice that it is tight and elastic, like the surface of a balloon. Unfortunately as we age, our skin thins and becomes loose and inelastic. Over time, muscle tension in the face becomes stronger than the skin's elasticity, and muscle contractions begin to create wrinkles. That's why when the muscles are paralyzed by injections of nerve toxins (such as botulinum toxin), the muscle tension is relaxed and the skin's elastic properties again predominate, producing a reduction or removal of wrinkles. However, those who are injected with the toxin still have biologically old skin. The only difference is, their muscles are now paralyzed. This is not aging reversal.

In contrast, the natural wrinkle-reduction methods described in this book restore the skin's thickness and elasticity; essentially transforming it into biologically younger skin. Removing damaged and cross-linked skin proteins, by replacing these proteins with new elastin and collagen and increasing the water-holding proteoglycans and glycosaminoglycans, produces a better moisturized and firmer skin. The SRCPs in creams or serums, such as those made by Skin Biology, have been shown to produce these effects. As previously noted, many of Skin Biology's products work even better when combined with hydroxy acids.

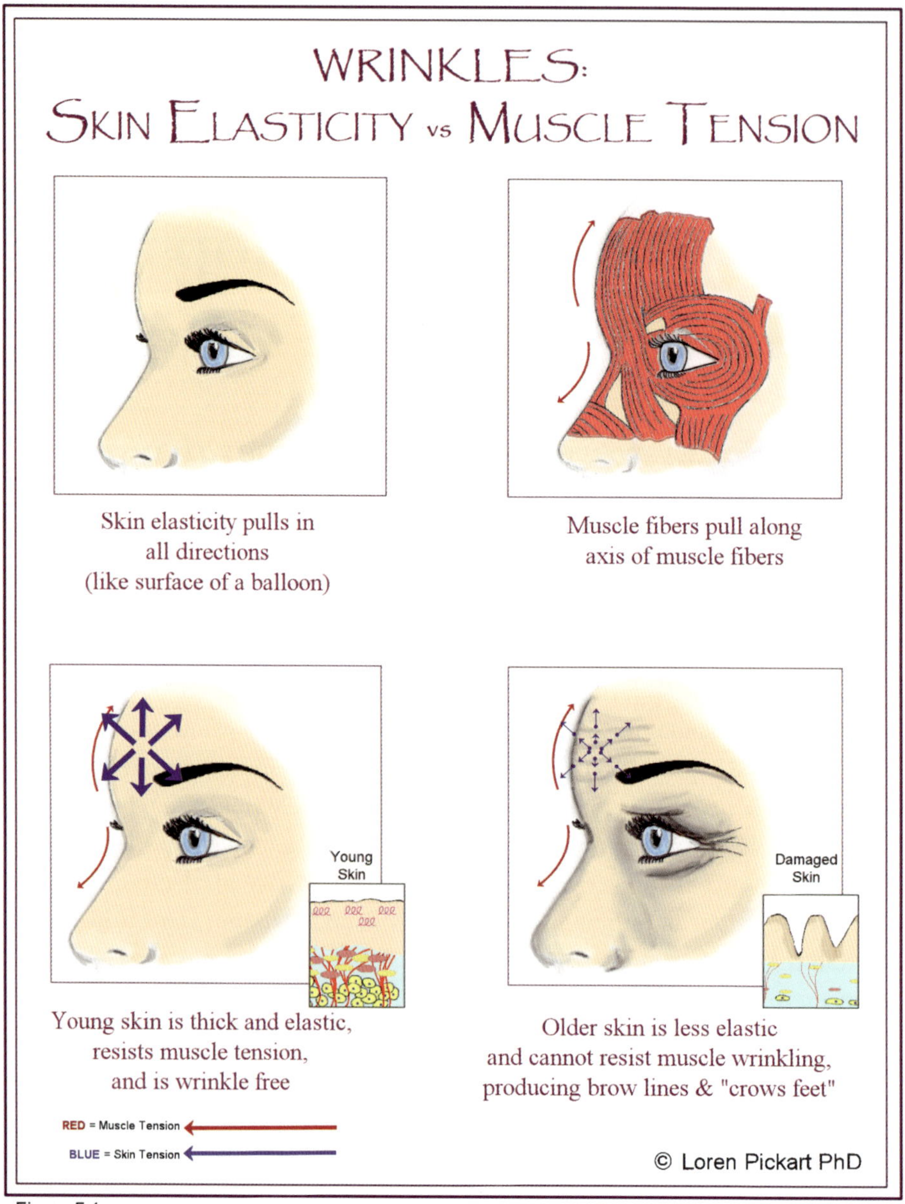

WRINKLES:
SKIN ELASTICITY vs MUSCLE TENSION

Skin elasticity pulls in all directions (like surface of a balloon)

Muscle fibers pull along axis of muscle fibers

Young skin is thick and elastic, resists muscle tension, and is wrinkle free

Older skin is less elastic and cannot resist muscle wrinkling, producing brow lines & "crows feet"

RED = Muscle Tension
BLUE = Skin Tension

© Loren Pickart PhD

Figure 5.1

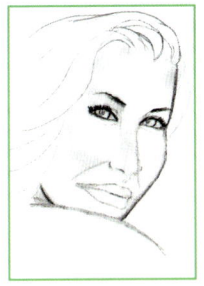

REMOVING WRINKLES
USING EXFOLIATING HYDROXY ACIDS and SRCPs (Natural Method)

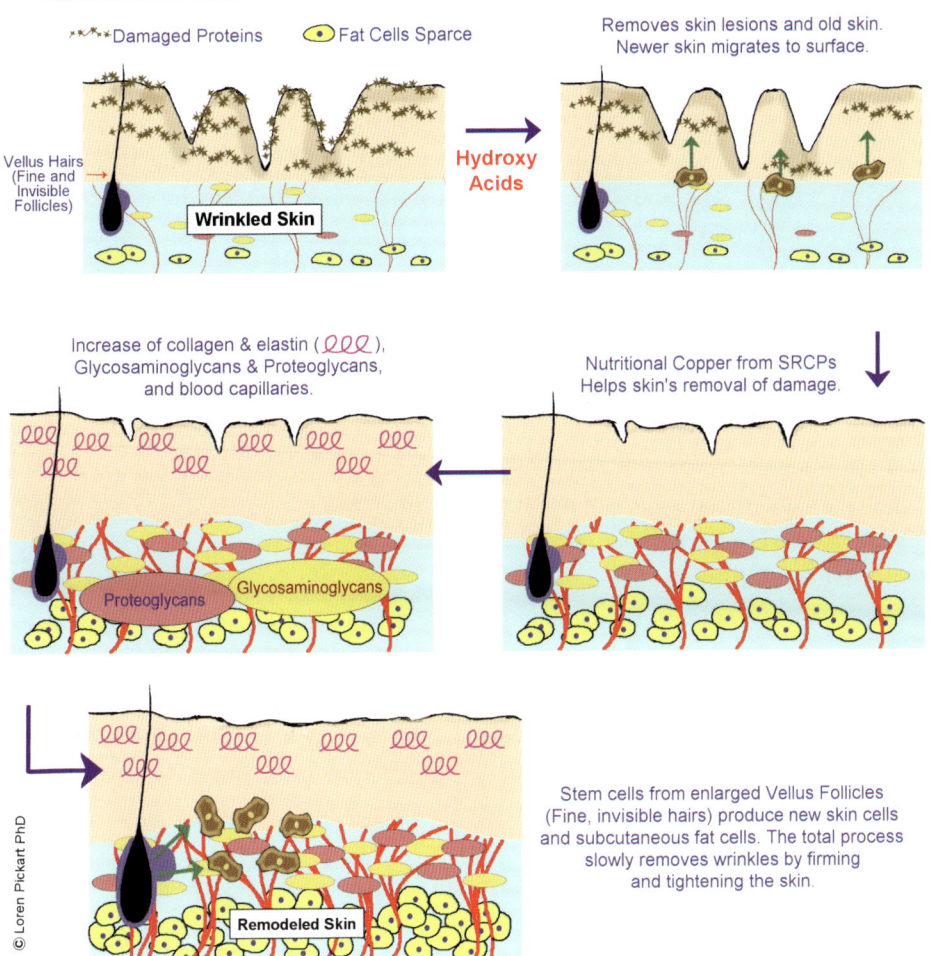

⁕⁕⁕ Damaged Proteins   ◯ Fat Cells Sparse

Vellus Hairs (Fine and Invisible Follicles)

Wrinkled Skin

Hydroxy Acids

Removes skin lesions and old skin. Newer skin migrates to surface.

Increase of collagen & elastin (ℓℓℓ), Glycosaminoglycans & Proteoglycans, and blood capillaries.

Proteoglycans   Glycosaminoglycans

Nutritional Copper from SRCPs Helps skin's removal of damage.

Remodeled Skin

Stem cells from enlarged Vellus Follicles (Fine, invisible hairs) produce new skin cells and subcutaneous fat cells. The total process slowly removes wrinkles by firming and tightening the skin.

© Loren Pickart PhD

Figure 5.2

Not all wrinkles are the same. There are two major types of wrinkles on the face, and wrinkle reduction must be handled differently for each. The first type of wrinkle includes the lines on the forehead, around the mouth, on the cheeks, and at the edge of the eyes (known as crow's feet). The other type of wrinkle is the lines around the eyes; these require special care, because the skin around the eyes is very thin and often has been damaged.

Treating Facial Wrinkles

The first type of wrinkle is reduced by alternating the use of hydroxy acids, which remove the skin in need of renewal, that is, the older layers of skin on the upper layer and by using SRCPs, such as Protect & Restore and Super Cop. The stronger hydroxy acids are more effective, however, many people find them irritating. When strong hydroxy acids are applied to the skin, a rash may develop or peeling may occur when the upper layer of the skin is removed by the strong acid concentrate. In general, it is better to use lighter, less concentrated hydroxy acids for a longer period of time.

Treating Wrinkles Around the Eyes

As the thinnest skin on the body, the skin surrounding the eyes is one of the most difficult areas to repair and keep healthy and young looking. This delicate skin is often chronically irritated and may be in a condition of sub-clinical inflammation. Years of using color cosmetics and other make-up, which contain a high concentration of dyes and metal salts, can produce extensive skin damage and sagging. In addition, cleansers used to remove make-up can cause further irritation by stripping away protective lipids from the skin.

Through Skin Biology's clients, I have discovered that using a progressively stronger remodeling system is the best way to treat the skin around the eyes. Most clients start with CP Night Eyes Premier (a relatively weak cream), then progress to CP Night Eyes Regular. When the skin adjusts to the SRCPs and becomes somewhat thicker and more protective, most clients move on to using Super CP Serum, and then finally to Super Cop. The last two are strong products that must be used gradually at first and at low concentrations.

If a client experiences irritation from using a Skin Biology product, I suggest that he or she use a biological healing oil to slow the uptake of the product. Applying either Emu Oil-S or Squalane before the SRCP product will result in a much milder response. You will recall that if you apply a BHO after a SRCP product instead, the oil will push more of the SRCPs into the skin and intensify their effect. In this manner, it is possible to adjust the SRCP action to receive maximum results. In general, hydroxy acids, even at a very low concentration, should not be used around the eyes.

When you first begin treating the delicate skin around the eyes, following these tips will help you adjust to your new regimen:

—Start by cleaning around the eye area to remove make-up. Use a very mild make-up remover such as Emu Oil-S for Skin, Squalane, or Gentle Clean liquid cleanser. Rinse the skin with clear water. Apply CP Night Eyes while the skin is still wet.

—Because the skin may be badly damaged, start with a very light coating of CP Night Eyes Premier, and then gradually increase the amount applied with time. If you experience irritation, that means too much copper peptide is passing through a very damaged skin barrier. A gentler approach is to use Emu Oil-S one night to replenish the skin lipids and CP Night Eyes every second night. (Some people discover that CP Serum is milder on damaged skin).

—As your skin barrier is repaired, you will become less sensitive to any applied product. With time, the skin around your eyes should tighten and firm and you can progress to more powerful products.

—If you experience excessive dryness, use a little less of the SRCP product and cover it with a light amount of either Emu Oil-Skin or Squalane.

Client Testimonials

Be patient when using SRCP products. Rebuilding the skin, particularly the delicate skin around the eyes, takes time, but eventually you will notice a difference. In some cases, your skin will look worse before it begins to look better. But don't just take my word for it. Read on to discover what Skin Biology's clients have to say.

From a client - first message:
I took a look at my eyes first thing this morning and man, I got to tell you, they looked awful! Big drooping, puffy half-moon ring underneath both of them. Much worse than the day before. At this time I look 100 percent worse than I did when I started CP Night Eyes two weeks ago. This is not good, but I haven't lost hope or faith in your products, I'm just concerned about what is happening and what I should do now. It would be nice to think that the puffiness is part of a reconstruction process going on under the outer skin. Is that possible? Are the effects of your products transdermal?

Same client - one week later:
My eyes are much better now! The puffiness is gone! I believe it was some deep rebuilding of the subdermal skin. The areas underneath my eyes are now filled out. I still have lots of small lines around the eyes, but I'm sure that the lines will vanish in time with continued use of your products. All and all a good experience using your product.
Thanks!
G.A., Washington

TIGHTEN AROUND THE EYES
(Total process may take 6-12 months)

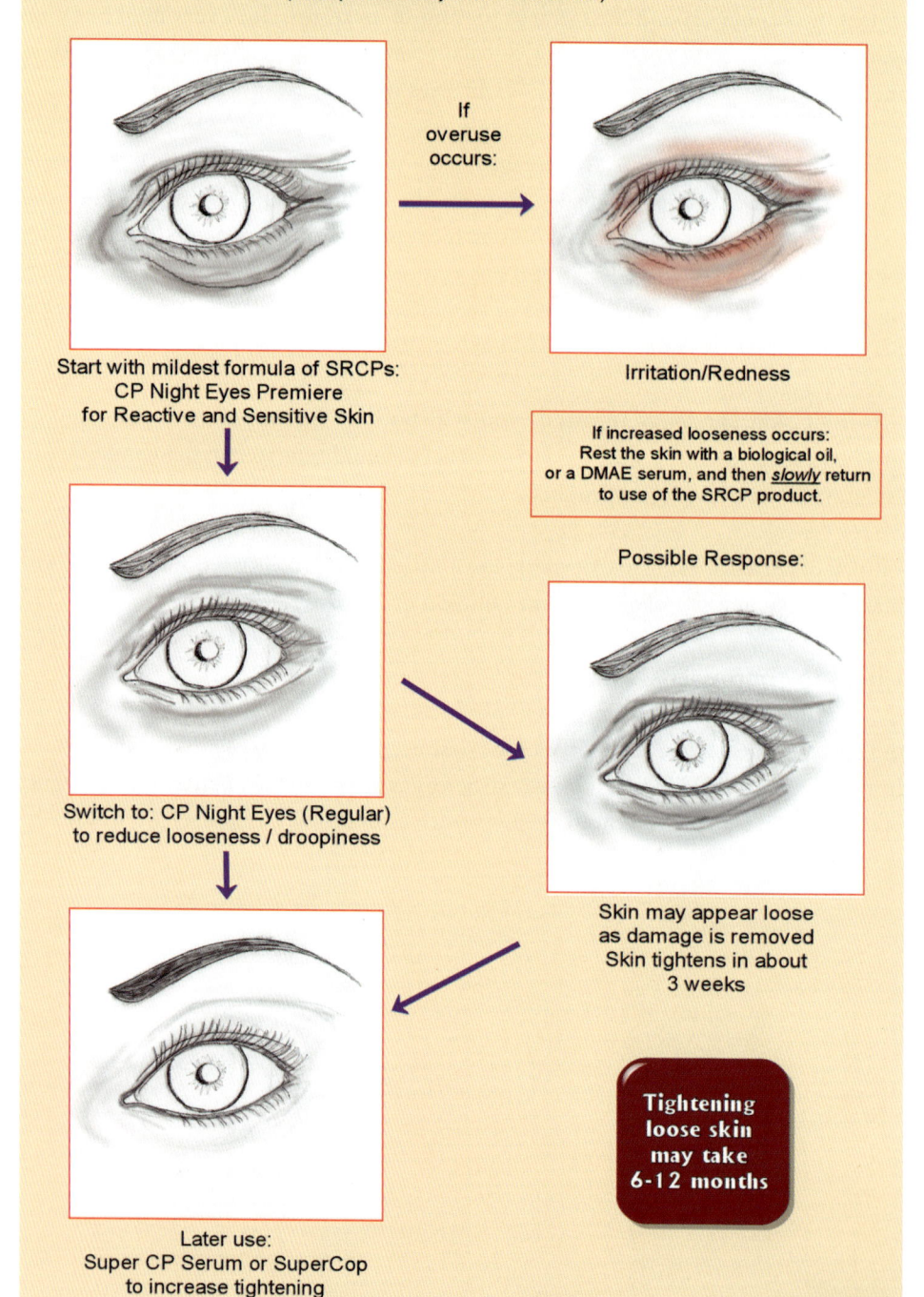

Start with mildest formula of SRCPs:
CP Night Eyes Premiere
for Reactive and Sensitive Skin

If overuse occurs:

Irritation/Redness

If increased looseness occurs:
Rest the skin with a biological oil,
or a DMAE serum, and then *slowly* return
to use of the SRCP product.

Possible Response:

Switch to: CP Night Eyes (Regular)
to reduce looseness / droopiness

Skin may appear loose
as damage is removed
Skin tightens in about
3 weeks

Later use:
Super CP Serum or SuperCop
to increase tightening

Tightening
loose skin
may take
6-12 months

Figure 5.3

TESTIMONIALS & EXPERIENCES:

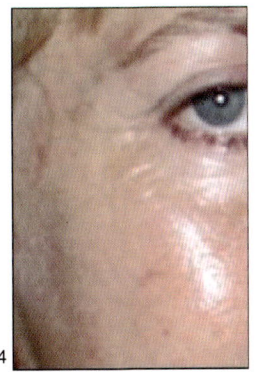

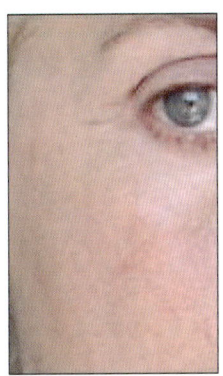

Figure 5.4

"I began working with Dr. Pickart's copper peptides consistently around November 2001...The changes in my skin within six months were just pretty unbelievable to me. I continued working with CP Serum, Exfol Serum and lots of oil. I began to introduce the Exfol cream to try to speed that sloughing off of the leathery old damaged cells that were migrating to the surface.

Quite evident [in the two pictures] is the reduction in wrinkles and crows feet. The discoloration during May 2002 was as a result of the copper peptides literally pushing or causing the damaged skin cells to migrate to the surface where they finally began to slough off. The sun-damaged spots are either gone or diminished greatly in size."

—Courtesy of Diana Yvonne (www.dianayvonne.com)

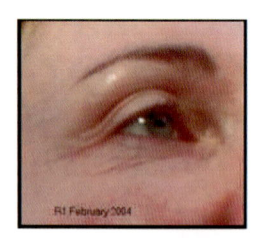

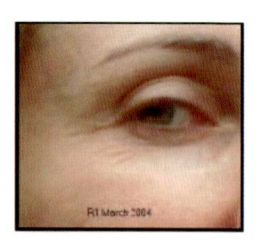

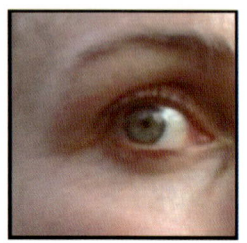

Figure 5.5

"Age 43: In November 2003, I introduced CP Night Eyes and I noticed two things: 1) the scales disappeared and 2) a little pin-prick-sized red mark that I'd had under my right eye for months and months was disappearing!

In comparing the progress pictures, the lid appears to have tightened up a lot. In the latest picture, looking down at the camera, the lines should be much more evident under the eye than when looking up as in the first photo. The dynamic smile lines are smoothing out fast along with the long one that ran underneath my eye are almost gone!"

—Submitted by R.
Courtesy of Diana Yvonne (www.dianayvonne.com)

Figure 5.6 — 26th may 2004 / 5th july 2004 / 25th july 2004 / 2nd oct 2004

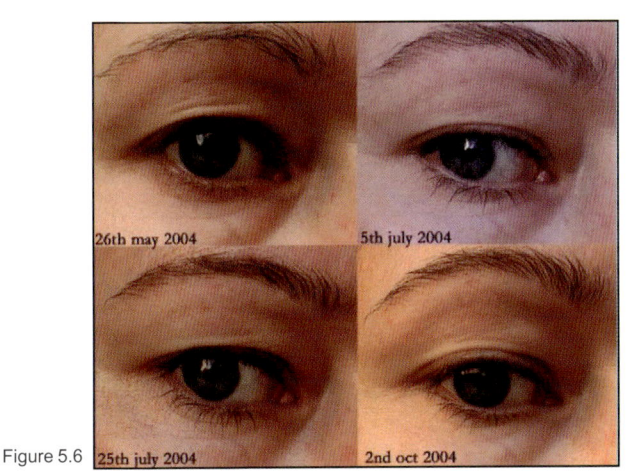

"I introduced CP Serum on May 26, 2004. I used it diluted the first night and felt no irritation. So I tried it full strength the second night (four drops for the entire face including around the eyes). As everything went fine, I've been using it undiluted since then. But I must say that my skin is really tough and that most people should really work their way up slowly. I currently only use CP Serum at night. In the last two months, the only new products I've included in my routine are: CP Serum, Exfol Cream and one 40 percent lactic peel weekly."

—Submitted by V.
Courtesy of Diana Yvonne (www.dianayvonne.com)

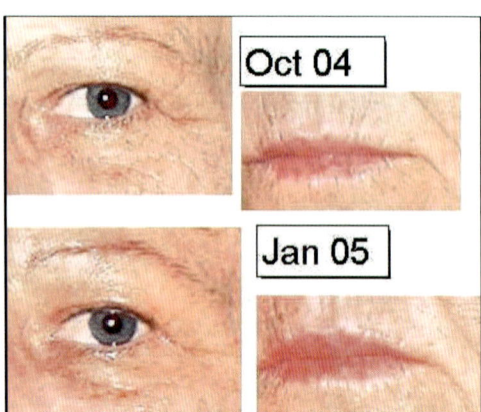

Figure 5.7

"I've only been using SkinBio for six weeks and glycolic since October 2004 (three months). Even I was surprised at the results I see here. The eyelid is much more visible and the major line at the corner of my eye is much softer. Of the two lines directly under my eye, one is now much less noticeable as well as the line near my eyebrow and above. Seems to me that my brow has lifted a little (not sure). The major lines are also much softer around my mouth. The texture of my skin is much better.

I saw two milia disappear from my eyelid I have had for weeks if not months. It [my skin] used to be blotchy and bumpy with occasional small breakouts (nothing serious). All these things have settled and my skin looks and feels much nicer. I cleanse well, apply 10 percent LA [lactic acid] and leave it on five minutes or so, and then wash it off in the shower. Before bed I apply exfol [Exfol Serum], wait anywhere from 10 to 30 minutes, and then apply CP Serum and Night Eyes, wait and then apply Emu Oil-S for Skin."

—Submitted by L.L.

Recommended Skin-Care Regimens

      The following are the anti-wrinkle and damage-removal regimens I recommend for three types of people: those under age 30 (and those over age 30 who have very oily skin); those over age 30 (and those under age 30 who have very dry skin); and those with rosacea.

For Those Under Age 30

1. In the morning after cleansing, apply a light amount of CP Serum. If acne is a problem, use Super CP Serum.

2. At night, apply Protect & Restore Classic Cream over your face three nights weekly and Exfol Serum three alternate nights weekly.

3. If dry patches are a problem, use Emu Oil-S. This does not cause breakouts.

For Those Over Age 30

1. In the morning after cleansing, apply a light amount of CP Serum, and then a light coating of Emu Oil-S or Squalane.

2. At night, apply Protect & Restore with Retinol over your face three nights weekly and Exfol Cream three alternate nights weekly.

3. After two months, you may progress to stronger hydroxy acids, such as a 30 percent lactic acid and Super Cop Cream. Be sure to use stronger products lightly at first.

For Those with Rosacea

1. In the morning after cleansing, apply a light amount of CP Serum followed by Emu Oil-S Lipid Replenisher.

2. At night, apply Protect & Restore Classic Cream over your face three nights weekly.

3. Sometimes Exfol Serum also helps to reduce rosacea. Apply the product lightly at night when not using Protect & Restore Classic Cream.

4. Gentle Clean cleanser works very well on the super-sensitive skin with rosacea.

Figure 5.8 Before 1st Face Lift

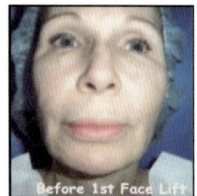

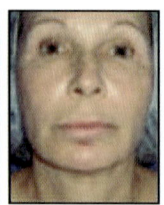

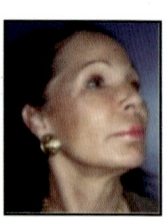

1. In the first step, the patient's face receives a treatment of microdermasion. Microdermabrasion gently abrades the face with professional grade crystals that are simultaneously vacuum removed.

2. The second step is an intermitting vacuum technique that results in an improved skin tone that helps reduce fine lines and wrinkles. The treatment starts at the lower areas of the neck first, then moves upward until all areas from forehead to chest have been effectively treated.

3. The client is then treated with skin remodeling copper peptide (SRCP) mask.

—Courtesy of Anti-Aging Clinic (www.anti-agingcliniccpc.com)

USING: Dermabrasion

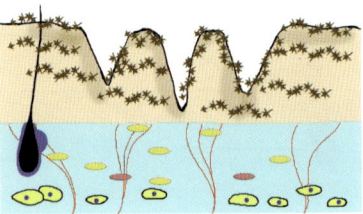

Dermabrasion with abrasive material smoothes top layer of skin

Dermabrasion performed on the skin

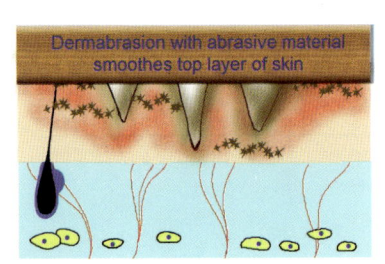

BETTER RESULT:
Follow with SRCPs and dermabrasion results in less redness and better healing.

SRCPs help activate the stem cells from enlarged vellus follicles to produce new skin cells and subcutaneous fat cells. Total process slowly firms and tightens skin after dermabrasion procedure.

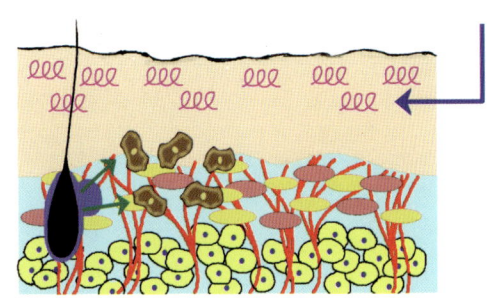

USING: Laser Resurfacing

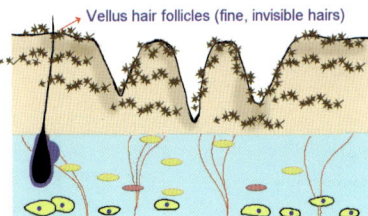

Damaged proteins   Few fat cells
Vellus hair follicles (fine, invisible hairs)

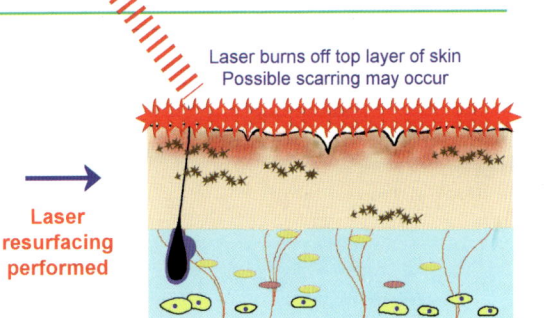

Laser burns off top layer of skin
Possible scarring may occur

Laser resurfacing performed

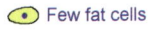

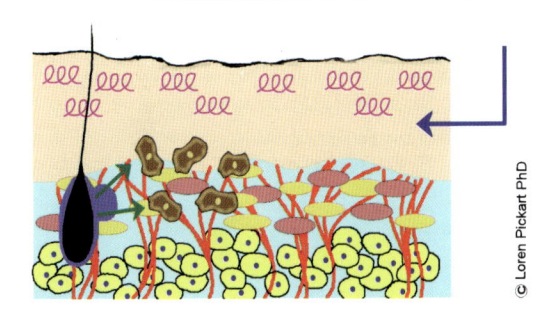

BETTER RESULT:
Follow with SRCPs and laser resurfacing results in fewer scars, less redness, and faster healing time.

SRCPs help activate the stem cells from enlarged vellus follicles to produce new skin cells and subcutaneous fat cells. Total process slowly firms and tightens skin after laser resurfacing procedure.

Figure 5.9

© Loren Pickart PhD

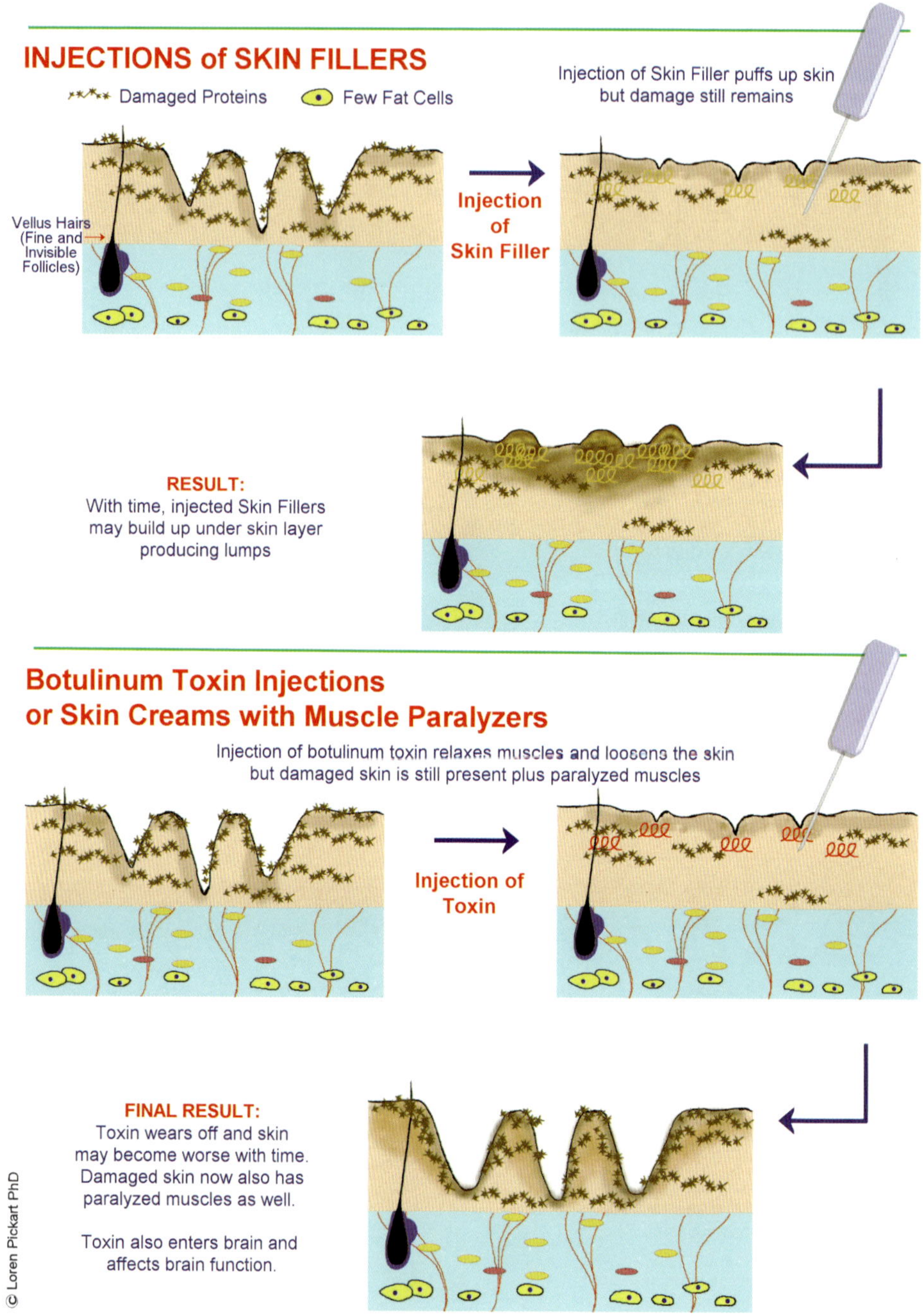

INJECTIONS of SKIN FILLERS

✶ Damaged Proteins   ⊙ Few Fat Cells

Injection of Skin Filler puffs up skin but damage still remains

Vellus Hairs (Fine and Invisible Follicles)

Injection of Skin Filler

RESULT:
With time, injected Skin Fillers may build up under skin layer producing lumps

Botulinum Toxin Injections or Skin Creams with Muscle Paralyzers

Injection of botulinum toxin relaxes muscles and loosens the skin but damaged skin is still present plus paralyzed muscles

Injection of Toxin

FINAL RESULT:
Toxin wears off and skin may become worse with time. Damaged skin now also has paralyzed muscles as well.

Toxin also enters brain and affects brain function.

© Loren Pickart PhD

Figure 5.10

Chapter 6

Tighten Loose and Sagging Skin

The Benefits of Biological Skin Tightening

One of the questions I hear most often from clients is how to fix the loosening of the skin that occurs with age. Loose or excessive skin can also plague those who have lost a significant amount of weight. A dermatologist or plastic surgeon might recommend surgery to fix this common problem, but there are many factors that make surgery a less-than-ideal option. Skin-tightening surgery is painful, expensive, and calls for a long recovery period. You can expect to wait at least a year before your rebuilt skin is fully recovered.

Most people would agree that a more appealing approach is to use the body's natural systems to tighten the skin. My goal in this book is to help you do so.

The most visible example of the body's natural skin-tightening process can be seen in the healing of wounds. Think of accidents in the kitchen, a small cut on the hand; afterward, you put a bandage on the wound. After a very short time, perhaps a few days, the wound is closed. Often during the healing process, the skin-tightening action is so intense that you can see stress lines on the skin as it pulls the sides of the wound together.

What pulls the skin together? Wounds are closed by two mechanisms. One is the rebuilding of tissue within the wound area. The second is the contraction of the skin around the wound. The use of SRCPs can enhance this process. In my work with SRCPs, one of my first discoveries was that they have a profound effect on tightening wounds. Often, when skin ulcers on hospital patients were treated with SRCPs, we would see strong wound contraction within 48 hours and the development of stress lines in the skin due to the intense pulling on the skin by the tightening of collagen strands.

Skin Wound Contraction & SRCPs

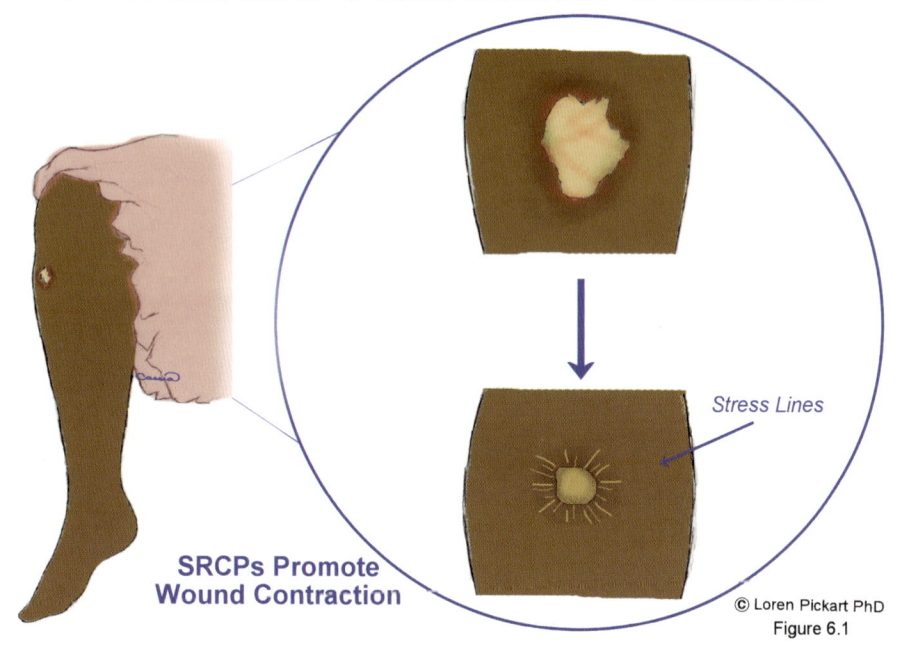

SRCPs Promote Wound Contraction

Stress Lines

© Loren Pickart PhD
Figure 6.1

The Natural Way to Tighten Skin

Think of young skin as the surface of a balloon; push it in or pull it out and it quickly returns to a smooth surface. Like the balloon, biological skin tightening occurs as the skin's repair cells, the fibroblasts, pull collagen strands together. Then collagen strands are biochemically attached to each other by the fibroblasts. This natural skin tightening keeps the skin elastic and soft. The fibroblasts use an enzyme called lysyl oxidase to connect the collagen strands, which requires both copper (II) and vitamin C to work.

As a result, adequate levels of copper (II) and vitamin C are essential for skin tightening. You can't get a tightening effect without having a high level of each in your skin. Copper (II) is best supplied from SRCPs applied to the surface of the skin. Vitamin C levels in the skin are easily increased by taking at least 1 gram daily as a supplement. It is difficult to get vitamin C through the skin except at a very low pH of about 2.5.

Biological Skin Tightening

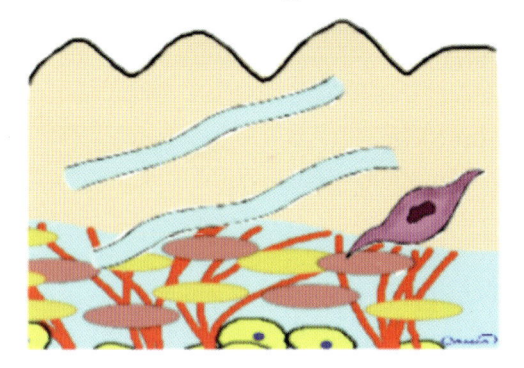

Collagen strands in loose skin:

SRCPs can help activate fibroblasts:
Attach to collagen strands, and as they contract, collagen strands are pulled closer and are chemically attached...

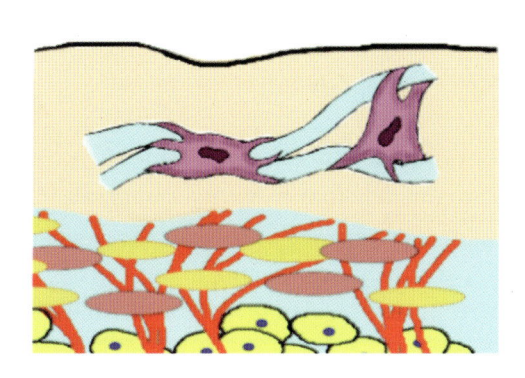

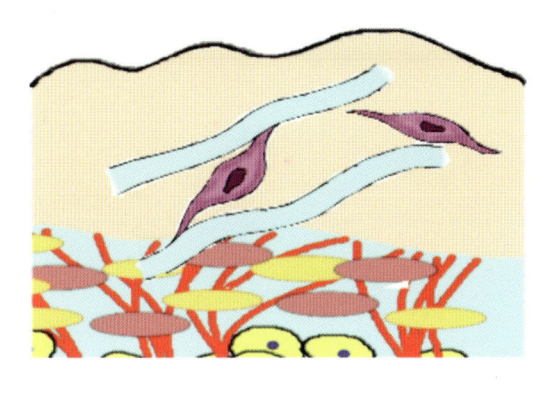

RESULT:
Tightened skin with elastic collagen that retains natural elasticity.

Figure 6.2

© Loren Pickart PhD

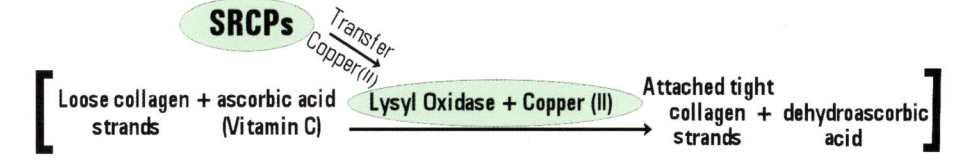

$$\left[\text{Loose collagen} + \text{ascorbic acid} \xrightarrow[\text{Lysyl Oxidase + Copper (II)}]{\text{SRCPs Transfer Copper(II)}} \text{Attached tight collagen} + \text{dehydroascorbic acid} \right]$$

The use of hydroxy acids, such as salicylic acid and lactic acid, also helps tighten the skin. Hydroxy acids remove the older cells on the skin's surface by producing a very mild skin damage. This damage assists in the skin renewal process, probably by increasing the number of fibroblasts.

Recommended Regimen for Tighter Skin
The following regimen has helped many Skin Biology clients turn back the clock on their skin:

1. Use SRCP products, vitamin C supplements (1 gram daily), and hydroxy acids to tighten the skin. Be patient; this is a slow process that takes several months, and the hydroxy acids can produce a mild irritation. Many clients use Exfol Cream in the morning and a strong SRCP cream (such as TriReduction with Retinol or Super Cop) at night. Some clients, after losing a large amount of weight, have used this procedure to avoid surgical removal of excess skin.

2. For maximum effectiveness, some clients apply a SRCP cream and a hydroxy acid at approximately four to six-hour intervals. Each product is used twice daily.

3. To speed things up, you might use a stronger hydroxy acid, such as a 15 percent to 30 percent lactic acid or glycolic acid. Mild microdermabrasion can also help you see faster results.

4. Take a daily supplement of 1 gram methylsulfonylmethane (MSM), which supplies the nutritional sulfur needed for the production of skin proteins.

Figure 6.3 — BEFORE / AFTER

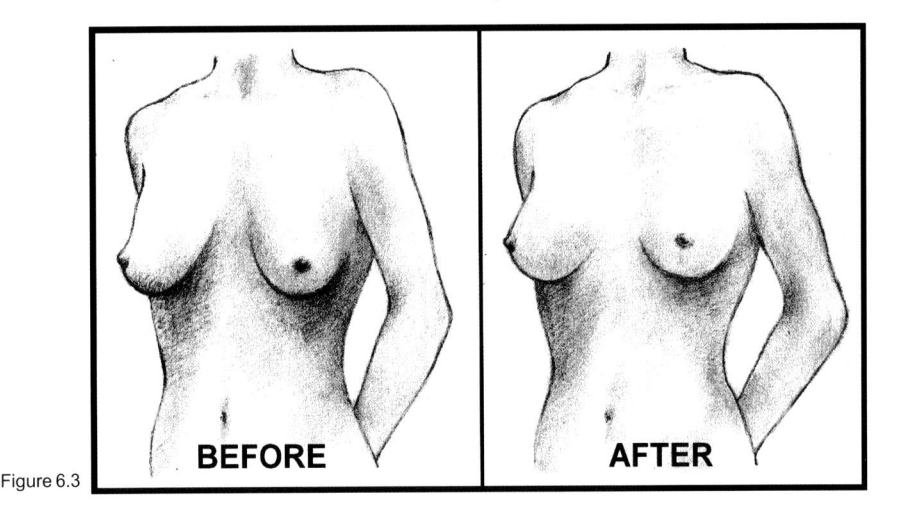

A slight breast lift can also be achieved by following this regimen. For this purpose, the best products to use are the Protect & Restore BND Cream and a 15 to 30 percent lactic acid or glycolic acid. Some women who were planning a surgical breast lift found this mild method gave enough improvement to satisfy them without surgery.

Other steps you can take to optimize your skin's natural tightening systems are eating a healthy diet and exercising regularly. If you are overweight, dieting will have a tightening effect on the skin. Consider how people who have been starving for a long time never have areas of loose skin on the body; the body absorbs excess skin when it can't find enough nutrients in the diet. Regular aerobic exercise tightens the internal muscles and enhances the rebuilding process.

Using Controlled Heating Methods to Tighten Skin

To return to our kitchen example, if you've ever burned yourself on the stove, you may have noticed that the burn caused your skin to contract. In serious burns, the resulting skin contraction can be so severe that it acts as a tourniquet and stops blood flow into the area. Often the burned skin is cut open to relieve pressure and permit blood flow again.

By the same token, controlled heating of the skin with lasers, microwaves, and various types of lights produces a mild contraction of the skin that can be effective in skin tightening. However, these methods are far from perfect; they do not produce collagen and may actually damage the vellus hair follicles that produce stem cells for skin rebuilding.

Those who use a controlled heating method must take care to treat the skin properly after the procedure, as the effectiveness depends on the skin's post-damage regenerative response. Using CP Serum followed by Emu Oil-S, beginning one to two weeks after the procedure, will result in softer skin with rebuilt collagen and elastin and less scarring.

Destructive Skin Tightening

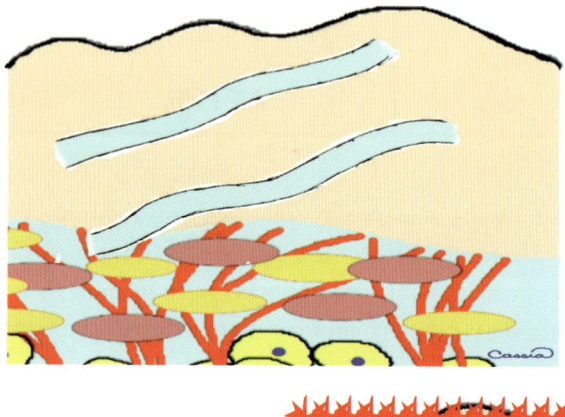

Collagen strands in loose Skin:

Destructive skin tightening methods denature collagen with heat, lasers, or other microwave devices...

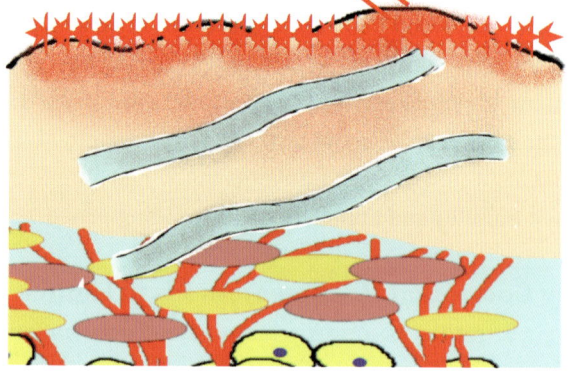

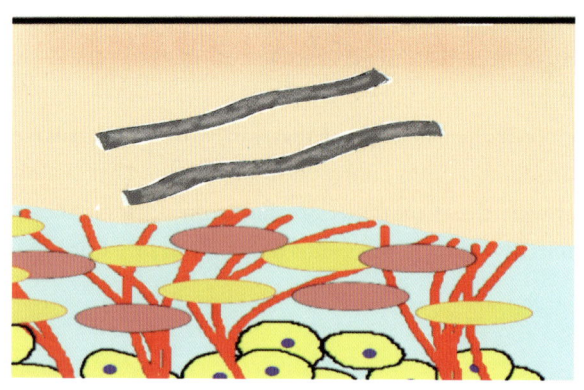

Collagen matrix shrinks like bacon in a pan, causing a general skin contraction.

RESULT: Tighter skin with condensed damaged collagen

© Loren Pickart PhD
Figure 6.4

SRCPs and Facial Resistance Training

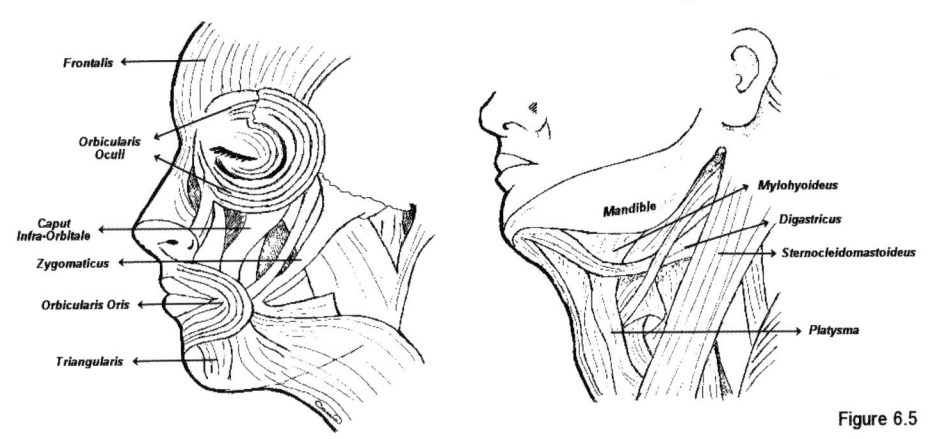

Figure 6.5

SRCPs increase the production of collagen and elastin, improving skin elasticity and firmness. However facial resistance training can prove beneficial in addition to this topical skincare regimen.

The skin and muscles in the face sag with time, but a regular applied program of facial exercise can help strengthen and lift, tone and tighten. Facial exercises create fullness and lift, especially in the cheeks, under the eyes, and around the chin and jaw. It fills in the hollows in the cheeks, flattens the areas under the eyes, and reduces sagging of the jowls, chin and neck area. The isometric, isotonic resistance training of FlexEffect can be successfully combined with SRCPs to achieve tighter, younger skin.

Information from FlexEffect (Facial Resistance Training: www.flexeffect.com)

Tightening Pores

Clogged and enlarged pores are a concern for many people. SRCPs and hydroxy acids can help to effectively reduce or tighten pores. Try the following:

1. In the morning, use a 2% salicylic acid pad (available at drugstores).

2. Apply a light amount of Exfol Serum and leave on the skin without washing off.

3. Apply a light amount of Super CP Serum (maximum of 4 drops daily when starting, then this amount can be slightly increased if needed). Additional suggestions include using pore cleansing strips every two weeks on problem areas and steam baths or saunas can also help with pore size reduction.

The Effect of SRCPs on Pores:

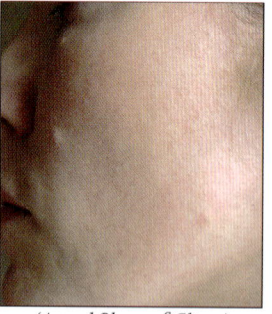

(Actual Photo of Client)

"I've been using Exfol, Protect & Restore, and Super Cop for over a year now, and have been meaning to write you for some time...Before I started using your products, I made a replica of my facial texture. Frankly, I was tired of wasting money on skin products that didn't perform as promised. I felt like my skin was softer and rosier right away. But then, over time, with good and bad days, I wasn't sure if I wanted to re-order. So, I made another facial texture replica and compared them side by side...I was so surprised at how much my skin texture had improved! Needless to say, I am using your products religiously, and I recommend them to friends...I am often complimented on my skin. I just wanted to let you know how nice it is to find an over the counter product that actually works, and can prove it!" – From Ohio, USA

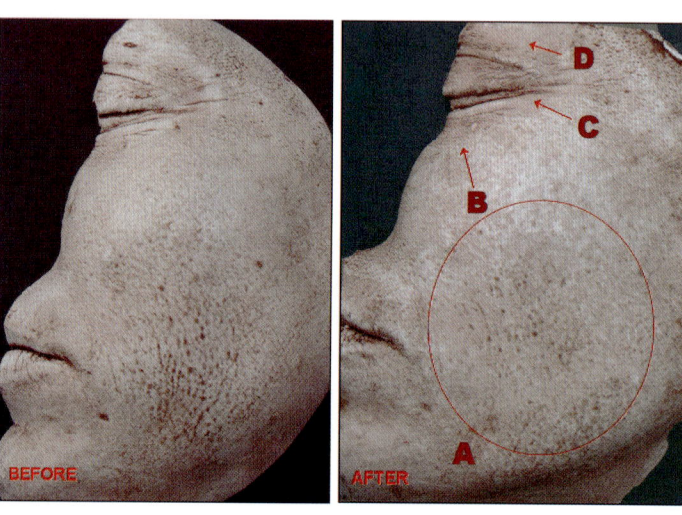

Figure 6.6

(Before and After of facial replica mask)

A Section of Face: Shows marked improvement in overall texture, tightened pores, and very visible reduced appearance of fine lines and spots.

B Section of Face: Look closely to see improvement of under eye skin area and skin health.

C Section of Face: Fine lines around eyelids have decreased and tightened. Notice additional lines of the eyelid area shown in the Before picture that are reduced in the After.

D Section of Face: Above eyelid area has improved in texture and loose skin has remodeled.

(Replicas are produced using indicator tint that highlights pores and intricate details of your skin. Find out more about Facial Replicas at www.plasticsurgerysculptures.com)

Testimonials on Tightening Pores:

"I have been using the Super Cop 2X on my enlarged pores on the nose (sparingly) and I have noticed in some of the areas they definitely appear to be smaller. I find it's great as my skin is oily and it doesn't make my nose any oilier either. Thank you so much!!!"
-K.N.

"Salicylic acid is lipid soluble and can deep cleanse the pores...My nose pores "disappeared" after three days, and the facial pores diminished after 1.5 weeks. My skin texture and pores continue to refine even after two months of using Exfol Serum and SRCPs. You could also add steam facials (add favorite herbs and citrus peels for added aromatherapy) for deep cleansing and refinement of pores."
-J.W.

"I have oily skin with large pores & have been using CP & Exfol Serums, Emu Oil or jojoba oil, & glycolic acid peels for about a year now. I've seen a definite difference in the size/appearance of my pores. They look smaller & are less noticeable - I don't know if it's because they are kept clear now or if they've actually tightened."
-G.B.

"The combination of keeping the pores clear with salicylic and the rebuilding of skin makes the pores look smaller...Try using Exfol twice a day and be sure to wait 30 minutes after applying it, before applying any other products. This will work on pore exfoliation."
-D.B.

"I have had great results using Exfol, Super CP Serum & Emu Oil, supplemented by 10% Lactic Acid and 5% BHA. The pores on my nose are improving everyday...I think the exfoliation is revealing pores that weren't noticeable because the skin had grown partially over them. And if skin had partially occluded the pore, that must be the reason why you could leave the house looking just fine and the next time you looked in a mirror there would be a pimple. I could never understand how it happened so fast, but when I think about it, it's almost like – how could you expect any other result. Those pores were ticking time bombs just waiting to mess up your world!"
-A.M.

> *We're all of us sentenced to solitary confinement inside our own skins, for life!*
> — Tennessee Williams

Chapter 7

The Balancing Act
For Removing Scars and Blemishes

How to Reduce Acne Scars and Other Blemishes and Help Your Skin Heal after Deep Peels, Laser Resurfacing, and Dermabrasion

If you suffered from acne as a teenager, you may have been left with unsightly acne scars as a reminder. These "minor skin imperfections," as they are often called, may seem minor in other people, but not when they appear on your own skin! Laser treatments and other methods commonly used to reduce acne scars and other skin blemishes aren't ideal—they are usually marginally effective, painful, expensive, and often produce further scars.

The good news is, surprisingly effective results can be achieved by using a combination of hydroxy acids and SRCPs. Treatment of this nature is low-cost and painless, although it may take several months to achieve optimal results.

> *CAUTION – These methods are not intended to replace regular skin care by a physician. Lesions that are dark and irregular, those that bleed, or are infected should be promptly checked by a physician.*

Skin blemishes occur when skin cells are re-programmed to grow in an abnormal manner after cellular damage from a variety of causes (viruses, bacteria, heat, UV or X-ray radiation, or incomplete wound healing that leaves scar tissue, etc). This abnormal skin must be removed so that normal healthy skin can re-fill the area and create smooth, unblemished skin. The key is to selectively remove the blemish as gently as possible while creating an environment that fosters the creation of new healthy skin.

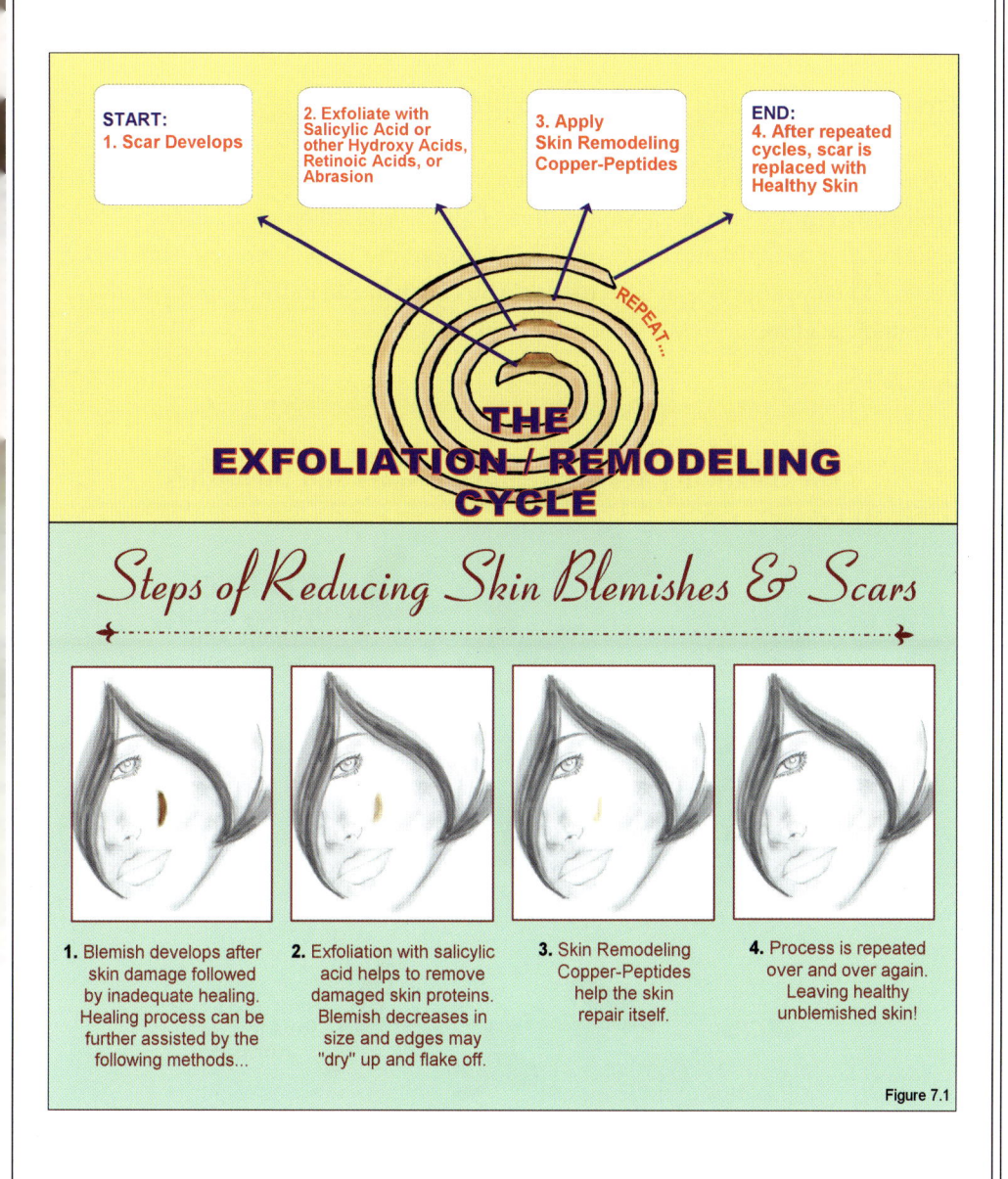

THE EXFOLIATION / REMODELING CYCLE

- **START:** 1. Scar Develops
- 2. Exfoliate with Salicylic Acid or other Hydroxy Acids, Retinoic Acids, or Abrasion
- 3. Apply Skin Remodeling Copper-Peptides
- **END:** 4. After repeated cycles, scar is replaced with Healthy Skin

REPEAT...

Steps of Reducing Skin Blemishes & Scars

1. Blemish develops after skin damage followed by inadequate healing. Healing process can be further assisted by the following methods...

2. Exfoliation with salicylic acid helps to remove damaged skin proteins. Blemish decreases in size and edges may "dry" up and flake off.

3. Skin Remodeling Copper-Peptides help the skin repair itself.

4. Process is repeated over and over again. Leaving healthy unblemished skin!

Figure 7.1

Most "old" dermatologists know that almost any skin lesion can be removed by the long-term application of hydroxy acids and/or retinoic acid or the use of liquid nitrogen. However, these approaches are limited by the strong skin irritation they cause. The skin lesion may be removed, but at the price of leaving a hole in the skin!

That's where SRCPs come in. SRCPs help calm and rebuild new skin, allowing skin lesions to be slowly dissolved and replaced by fresh, unblemished skin. In this chapter, you will discover how to use hydroxy acids and SRCPs to treat many common scars and help your skin heal after cosmetic procedures.

First Restore Health, Then Remove Blemishes

Often damaged skin is so fragile that it must be restored to better health before lesions can be removed with hydroxy acids and retinoic acid. So the first step in blemish removal is to use a combination of SRCPs and a biological healing oil, such as Emu Oil-S or Squalane, for two weeks to a month to help nurse your skin back to health. When your skin is in better shape, you can then add in the hydroxy acid and/or retinoic acid to speed skin-lesion removal.

The Balancing Act for Removing Scars and Blemishes

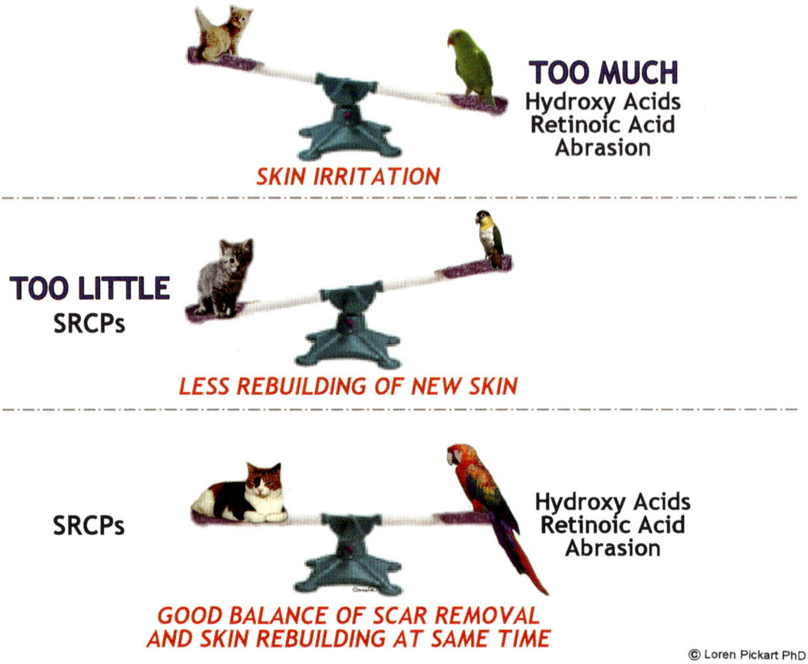

TOO MUCH
Hydroxy Acids
Retinoic Acid
Abrasion

SKIN IRRITATION

TOO LITTLE
SRCPs

LESS REBUILDING OF NEW SKIN

SRCPs — Hydroxy Acids
Retinoic Acid
Abrasion

GOOD BALANCE OF SCAR REMOVAL AND SKIN REBUILDING AT SAME TIME

Figure 7-2

© Loren Pickart PhD

The Balancing Act

Over years of observations, I found a number of routines that help remove many types of skin blemishes (scars and pitted scars, skin tags, moles, sun damage, stretch marks, warts, hyperpigmentation, discoloration, and so on). These often can be removed with repeated use of moderate-strength hydroxy acids and SRCPs. The hydroxy acids slowly loosen and dissolve the blemished tissue, while the SRCPs help rebuild new skin. This method is slow, but effective and does not cause excessive skin irritation.

For blemish removal, hydroxy acids are usually rubbed into the blemish area in the morning, followed by an SRCP product at night. The stronger hydroxy acids and Skin Biology products work faster, but irritation can sometimes be a problem with the stronger products, so they should be used with caution. Using retinoic acid and/or abrasion, such as dermabrasion, pumice stones, and needling (subcision), can also help speed the removal of blemishes.

The hydroxy acids and SRCPs work best when used every day. Some clients with severe scars have experienced good results by applying the products up to four times daily (for example, a hydroxy acid at 8 a.m., a SRCP product at noon, a hydroxy acid at 5 p.m., and a SRCP product before bedtime). You should see an improvement in about a month, but some old scars, such as stretch marks and keloid scars, may take six to eight months to slowly fade. Skin usually reverts to its pre-damage color.

When using strong hydroxy acids, your skin is more sensitive to sunlight, so use a sun protectant on your skin that contains a physical sunblocker such as pure titanium dioxide.

Remember, blemish removal is a balancing act. Too much removal of blemished skin produces a hole in the skin, while using too few SRCPs may be ineffective. Depending on your skin type and condition, you may have to use more or less of the blemish-reduction products. In general, it is best to go slowly. Your skin can only change and improve so fast.

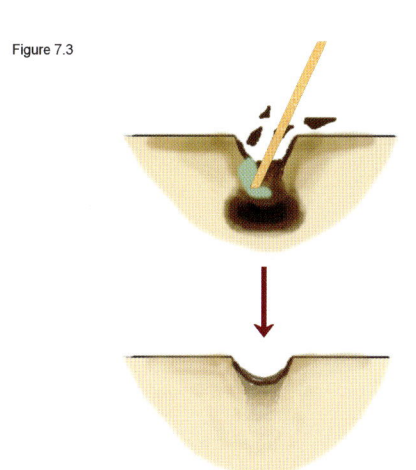

Figure 7.3

A toothpick or similar utensil can be used to apply the SRCPs directly to the area, and at the same time helps with light abrasion.

Skin Lesion Removal

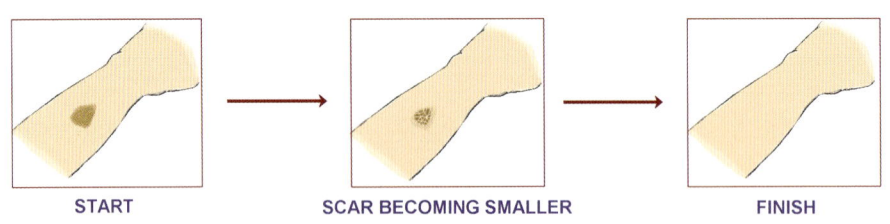

START → SCAR BECOMING SMALLER → FINISH

DIFFERENT TYPES OF SKIN LESIONS

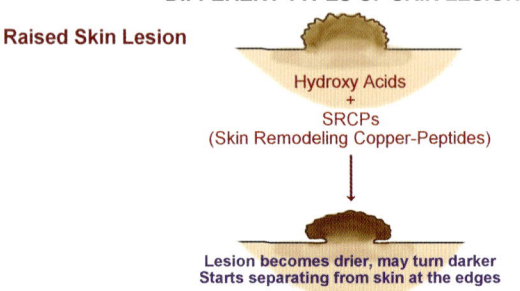

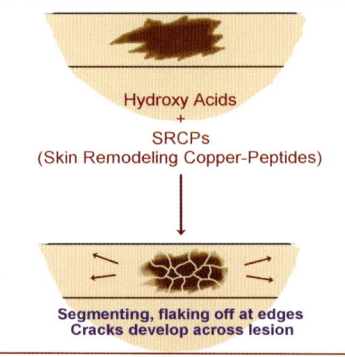

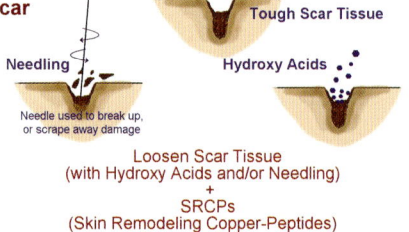

Raised Skin Lesion

Hydroxy Acids
+
SRCPs
(Skin Remodeling Copper-Peptides)

Lesion becomes drier, may turn darker
Starts separating from skin at the edges

Flat Skin Lesion

Hydroxy Acids
+
SRCPs
(Skin Remodeling Copper-Peptides)

Segmenting, flaking off at edges
Cracks develop across lesion

Pitted Acne Scar

Tough Scar Tissue

Needling — Hydroxy Acids

Needle used to break up, or scrape away damage

Loosen Scar Tissue
(with Hydroxy Acids and/or Needling)
+
SRCPs
(Skin Remodeling Copper-Peptides)

When performed over and over
Scar is removed and skin pulls itself flat

© Loren Pickart PhD

Figure 7.4

Depressed Scars:
Why Things May Appear to Look Worse
Before They Look Better

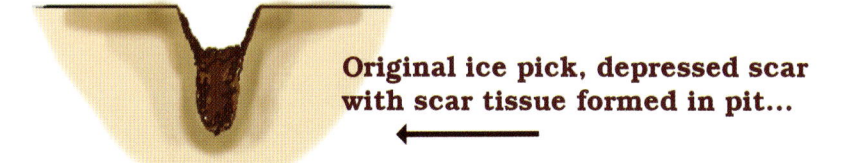

Original ice pick, depressed scar with scar tissue formed in pit...

Hydroxy Acids are applied and scar tissue begins to break up...

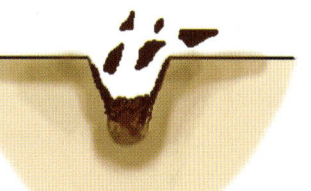

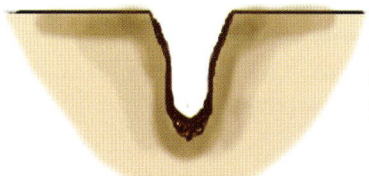

As scar tissue is removed, scar may become deeper for a time...

But this does not last, SRCPs help rebuild healthy skin and slowly the depressed area fills in!

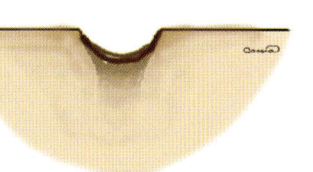

© Loren Pickart PhD

Figure 7.5

Layers of Damage:
Why Things May Appear to Look Worse Before They Look Better

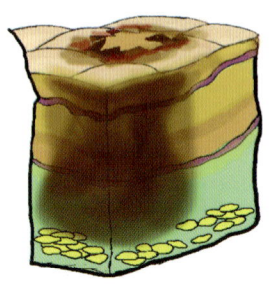

Damage from acne infection appears on top of Skin Layer, but reaches deep into skin...

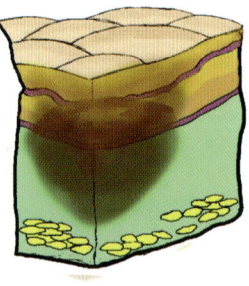

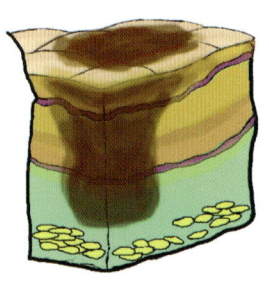

In time, skin may cover and hide damage but scar tissue still lies beneath...

As hydroxy acids + abrasion + SRCPs work on the skin, the damage that was below may be revealed...

But this does not last and as scar tissue is removed, Healthy Skin is revealed!

© Loren Pickart PhD

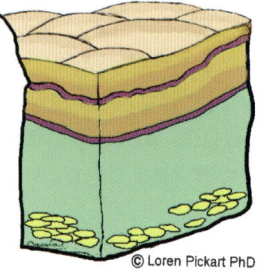

Figure 7.6

How Hydroxy Acids and SRCPs Work

Hydroxy acids, such as salicylic acid and lactic acid, are widely used as exfoliating agents and for skin peels. They remove dead skin cells and can also loosen and slowly dissolve skin lesions such as acne scars, skin tags, stretch marks, sun-damage marks, and moles.

The secret behind the hydroxy acids' action is that healthy, normal skin has a resistance to such acids and the damage they cause is quickly repaired with the aid of the SRCPs. Most skin lesions are less resistant to this treatment and slowly dissolve away. The irritation caused by the hydroxy acids may also activate some enzymes and immune cells that help remove damaged skin and lesions. As a result, using hydroxy acids over a period of a month or longer slowly dissolves most skin lesions and new unblemished skin rises to the surface. This is essentially a modification of normal skin-peel techniques where a very strong hydroxy acid (or other peeling agent such as TCA or phenol) is used.

Skin peels work well under perfect circumstances. However, they can be highly irritating if the subsequent regenerative response of the skin is inadequate to fully heal the acid-treated skin. In other words, if too little skin rebuilding takes place, the peeling agent may cause further scarring or inflammation. However, by using an SRCP product after the hydroxy acids, you create an environment that prompts the regeneration of normal, healthy skin. Hydroxy acids and SRCPs complement one another; while the repeated application of hydroxy acids slowly dissolves skin blemishes, SRCPs aid in the rebuilding of healthy, smooth skin. As the skin is rebuilt and scars are removed, the elastic properties of the skin pull it into a smooth surface.

Reduction of Acne Scars and Pitted Scars

For acne scar reduction, it is essential to avoid new breakouts. The following regimen has been found effective by many of Skin Biology's clients, both for preventing acne and reducing acne scars and other pitted scars. As with all scars and blemishes, the key is to be patient and keep working on the scar.

1. In the morning, wipe your face with a 2 percent salicylic acid pad (available at drugstores).

2. After the salicylic acid pad, apply a light amount of Exfol Serum (2 percent salicylic acid in a supportive liquid) and leave it on.

3. At night, apply Super CP Serum (a SRCP serum plus salicylic serum) and leave it on. Start with a maximum of four drops daily, and then slowly increase the amount.

4. For pitted scars, some people use stronger hydroxy acids and/or retinoic acid in the morning.

5. About every two weeks, use pore-cleansing strips (available at drugstores) on acne-prone areas. Be careful not to overuse the strips to the point of irritation.

6. Some people use this method one day and anti-acne products (such as benzoyl peroxide or Retin-A) on alternate days.

7. Anti-acne products and Super CP Serum can be somewhat drying to the skin. Emu Oil-S works well as a moisturizer and rarely increases breakouts.

Reduction of Skin Tags

Skin tags are small, generally benign skin growths. They often fall off naturally, and hydroxy acids are known to speed up their removal. Applying SRCPs also seems to help by aiding the recovery of normal skin around the skin tag.

The following regimen has been found effective by many of Skin Biology's clients. Some skin tags are more resistant than others, but you should see significant results in about a month.

1. In the morning, apply Exfol Cream (a beta hydroxy acid product) to the skin tag.

2. Apply more Exfol Cream during the day, but reduce the amount if your skin becomes irritated.

3. In the evening, apply TriReduction with Retinol, Super Cop, or Super Cop 2X to the skin tag.

4. You can also use the SRCP product in the morning, but because of the blue color, most people prefer evening use.

Sometimes the Exfol Cream's salicylic acid irritates the skin tag and it becomes reddened. If this happens, you may want to reduce the frequency of application, but try to find a schedule that allows you to keep applying the cream on a regular basis.

Reduction of Stretch Marks

Stretch marks arise when the skin is overextended. This often occurs during pregnancy or vigorous muscle building.

The following regimen has been found effective by many of Skin Biology's clients. It will take about a month before you notice an improvement, and really good results may take several months. Be patient; we have had reports from women saying they were able to remove stretch marks from pregnancy that were up to 30 years old!

1. In the morning, apply Exfol Cream to the stretch mark.

2. Apply more Exfol Cream during the day, but reduce the amount if your skin becomes irritated.

3. In the evening, apply TriReduction with Retinol to the stretch mark.

4. You can also use the SRCP product in the morning, but because of the blue color, most people prefer evening use.

Reduction of Sun Damage

Darkening of the skin due to sun damage and other sun-damage marks (actinic keratosis) can be markedly reduced or removed by using a combination of SRCPs and beta hydroxy products and/or retinol. Results should be evident in about a month as a reduction in the area and thickness of the lesion. After a week, you may notice a slight flaking of the skin around the periphery of the damage. This is usually followed by a shrinking and thinning of the lesion.

The following regimen has been found effective by many of Skin Biology's clients.

1. In the morning, apply the Exfol Cream to the sun-damage mark.

2. Apply more Exfol Cream during the day, but reduce the amount if your skin becomes irritated.

3. In the evening, apply the SRCP product to the sun-damage mark. The best products are TriReduction or Super Cop. Start with a light application. For the sensitive breast and décolletage area, use Protect & Restore for Breast, Nipples, and Décolletage.

4. You can also use the SRCP product in the morning, but because of the blue color, most people prefer evening use.

Reduction of Moles

Moles can be slowly reduced and often removed with mild hydroxy acids and copper peptides. However, faster results will be obtained with stronger products. Some skin clinics apply 70 percent glycolic acid to moles with a cotton-tipped swab for six minutes. This must be done by a skin-care expert. When the acid is washed off, a copper-peptide product such as CP Serum is applied. CP Serum is applied nightly at bedtime for a few more days. After this procedure, many moles drop off in two to three days' time.

If You Want Faster Results

With most of the skin-care regimens described so far, using stronger hydroxy acids will speed up the process. However, stronger hydroxy acids also increase the chances of irritation or chemical burns. The strongest Skin Biology product is 2 percent salicylic acid at pH 3.2. Some estheticians and clinics use 10 percent salicylic acid or 30 to 70 percent alpha hydroxy acids to loosen scar tissue, then apply the copper-peptide product. These stronger hydroxy acids can be obtained from estheticians and dermatologists or from the resellers in the Resource chapter.

Some clients use the types of pads (17% to 40% salicylic acid) and salicylic acid (12% to 17%) solutions that are used to remove calluses and warts. These work well on many types of skin lesions, but again be cautious and do not over use such products. The pads or solutions are applied at one time of the day, or on alternate days, and the SRCPs at a different time.

Skin Abrasion and Scar Reduction

Methods that mildly abrade skin, such as microdermabrasion and needling (subcision), are also useful in speeding scar reduction when combined with hydroxy acids and SRCPs. Some old scars are very hard and tough, and a physical breakdown of the scar through microdermabrasion, exfoliating wash cloths, pumice stones, or needling allows the hydroxy acids to start dissolving it. For elevated or flat scars, microdermabrasion works well. For depressed scars, such as pitted acne scars, subcision by an esthetician can be used to break up deeply buried scar tissue. In this procedure, a needle (similar to a tattoo needle) disrupts the scar collagen and stimulates its replacement by newly formed collagen. The best results are achieved with several sessions.

Some estheticians tell us that they use CP Serum or TriReduction after the needling and see a much better and faster clearing of the scar. However, do not apply the copper peptides until the wound has scabbed over and is no longer open or oozing liquid.

Post-Procedure Healing

After Peels, Laser Resurfacing, and Dermabrasion

In addition to reducing many types of scars, hydroxy acids and SRCPs can enhance healing after skin peels, laser resurfacing, and dermabrasion. The rest of this chapter will describe how to use hydroxy acids and SRCPs effectively during post-procedure recovery.

After a Chemical Peel

Chemical peels may produce severe irritation that leads to scars and prolonged redness. After a peel, some type of moisturizer and/or an anti-inflammatory to reduce irritation is usually applied. However, simple coverings such as petrolatum do not stop the development of redness and inflammation. A peel followed by cortisone used as an anti-inflammatory often defeats the purpose since the cortisone inhibits skin repair. So while the peel removes blemishes and dead skin, the subsequent skin rebuilding is inhibited. This can produce very thin skin.

SRCPs have anti-inflammatory actions that can help. Unlike cortisone, which inhibits skin repair, SRCPs enhance skin repair and inhibit the action of Interleukin-1, a cytokine that increases skin damage after injury, and TGF-ß-1, the scar-forming protein. After a chemical peel, some of our clients have experienced dramatic results by following these steps:

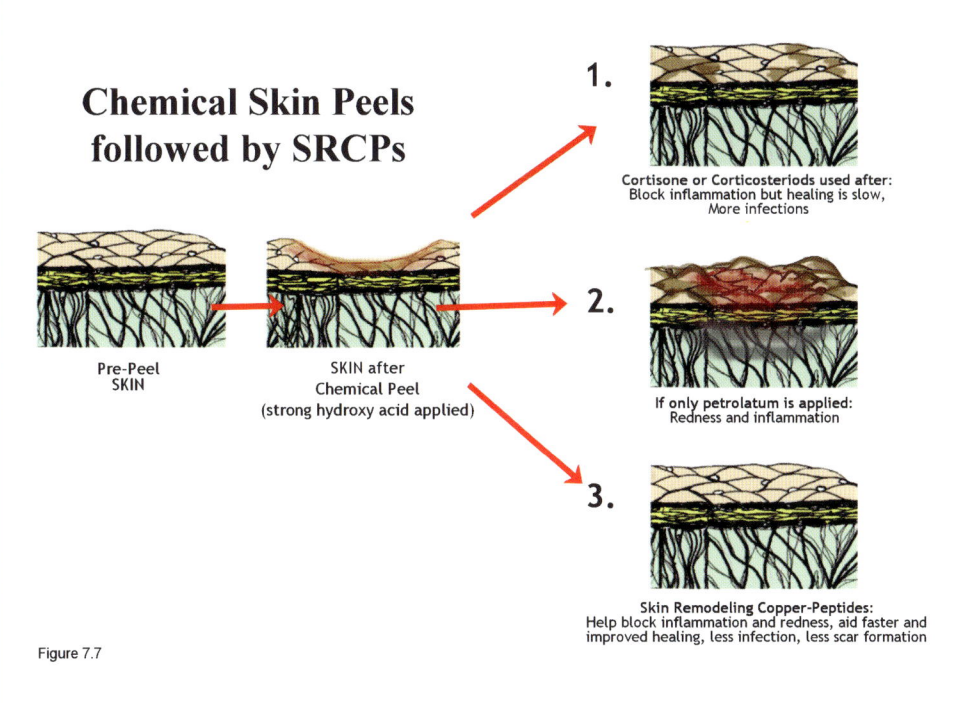

Figure 7.7

1. In hot climates, apply TriReduction Basic after the peel. This product contains SRCPs and high levels of squalane and octyl palmitate as skin protectants.

2. In cool climates, apply CP Serum followed by Emu Oil-S after the peel.

3. The first use of SRCP products should be within two hours of the peel, then on a twice-daily basis. Use the products lightly.

After Laser Resurfacing and Dermabrasion

Again, some of our clients have experienced dramatic results by following these steps.

1. Apply CP Serum to the skin within two hours of the procedure.

2. Apply a thin coating of CP Serum daily to the healing skin. Be careful to use only a light coating of CP Serum. Too often, people think more is better.

For Skin that Remains Irritated, Reddened, or Has New Scars

Often after a procedure such as a chemical peel, the treated skin is irritated and sore. Sometimes burns and hyperpigmentation marks are visible. This state can exist for a year or longer after the procedure. The following is a regimen that can help.

1. Apply Emu Oil-S until the soreness is alleviated.

2. When the soreness is gone, apply CP Serum followed by Emu Oil-S on a daily basis. Be careful to use only a light coating of CP Serum. A small amount of CP Serum is quite effective.

Skin recovery by this method is slow, but you should notice a significant improvement in a month. For severely burned or irritated skin, full recovery may take several months.

Rosacea

Often rosacea (The Curse of the Celts) can be controlled by the use of mild skin cleansers, such as Skin Biology's Gentle Clean, followed by CP Serum and Emu Oil-S.

Chapter 8

Special Concerns
When Make-up Ravages the Skin
For Models, Actors and Make-up Lovers

Have you ever watched a young actress on the movie screen and notice something strange about her skin? From afar, the actress appears to have a perfect complexion. But in close-up scenes, you notice that she actually has skin riddled with moles, spots, or other skin damage. How does this happen?

Many of the people who make it in show business start out with the best looks, including beautiful skin. Some actors and actresses even begin their careers as models before they end up on the big screen, and no doubt are successful in part due to their healthy, glowing complexion. But many things happen to change this along the way.

Challenges to be "Faced"

Acting and modeling are unique. Actors, actresses and models are constantly under scrutiny by the millions of people who see them on the screen and in magazines. No other occupations require the same dedication to upholding one's appearance (in body as well as skin) as do these two professions. Sadly, the lifestyle of actors and models—including the constant application and removal of make-up, the harsh effects of stage lighting and a high level of stress—often takes a toll on the skin. This is especially true for actresses and female models.

Special Concerns of Models/Actors

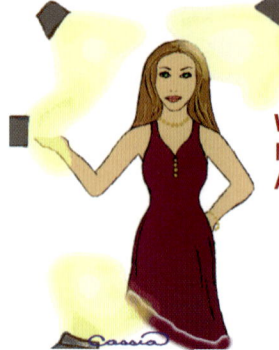

What are the special concerns of Models and Actors? There are many... And here is what SRCPs can do to help

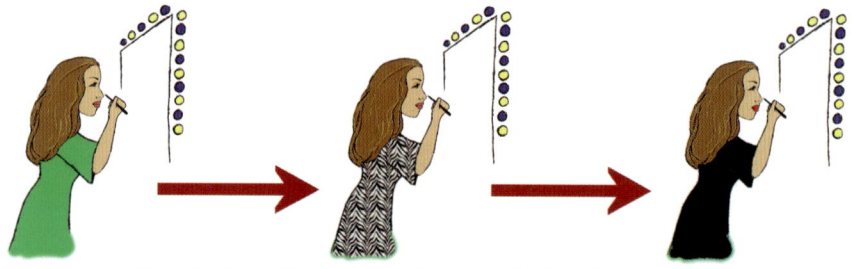

Constant applications and removal of makeup (with its colored salts and chemical dyes) and makeup removers (which damage both the protective acid mantle and the skin's protein/lipid barrier) are harsh on skin. Long hours of heavy makeup on the skin, scene changes and touch ups, lights used in the industry and the stress to keep skin looking blemish-free can take its toll.

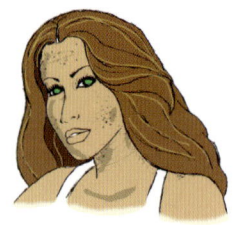

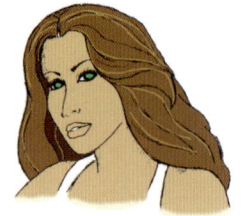

1. Before applying makeup, apply a very light protective layer of CP Serum.

2. Remove makeup with Emu Oil-S or Squalane.

3. Cleanse with Skin Biology's Gentle Clean Cleanser.

4. Repair your skin with CP Serum + Emu Oil-S.

5. Remove damage marks with Exfol Cream or Exfol Serum.

6. Repair with TriReduction Cream or stronger SRCPs:

Super Cop Cream or Super CP Serum

Figure 8.1

© Loren Pickart PhD

The most damaging factor that actors and models face is the constant application and removal of make-up. Both make-up (with its colored salts and chemical dyes) and make-up removers (which remove the protective acid mantle) are harsh on the skin. Make-up is often quickly applied, and then completely removed, followed by another color change (See dramatization). Other times, heavy make-up is worn for many hours at a stretch before being stripped away with a make-up remover at the end of the day.

Whatever the circumstances, the frequent application and removal of make-up makes the skin more susceptible to the development of skin damage, warts, moles, sun damage, and skin lesions. It is therefore essential for actresses and models to learn how to properly protect and care for their skin.

Skin-care Tips for Actors and Models
Here are some easy steps for actors and models to follow that are designed to address the specific concerns they face.

General Guidelines
1. Before applying make-up, use a Skin Biology serum or cream as a base to protect the skin. These products have been specially formulated for this purpose.

2. Hydroxy acids work well to remove dead skin cells and damaged skin proteins, dissolving damage that has become apparent on the skin.

3. In the morning, exfoliate with a beta hydroxy acid product such as Exfol Cream or Exfol Serum, which contain 2 percent salicylic acid. Apply the product lightly to the face or skin area.

4. In the evening, spot-treat damaged areas with TriReduction Cream following by Super CP Serum or Super Cop Cream. Generally, serums work best for combination or oily skin and creams for drier skin.

To Protect the Skin After Make-up Sessions

1. Use only biological healing oils to remove make-up. BHOs are much better for the skin than harsh chemical removers, which have a drying effect. Oils such as Emu Oil-S or Squalane work well.

2. To remove make-up, first apply a BHO lightly to the face, and then rub gently to remove the make-up. Finally, rinse thoroughly with warm water. Any remaining oil helps replenish the skin's natural oils.

3. After make-up is removed, follow with a mild cleanser. With a pH of 7.5, Skin Biology's Gentle Clean is a good one to use. Many soaps and cleansers not only remove surface dirt and oils, but actually damage the skin by destroying its natural protection imparted by the acid mantle and the skin's protein/lipid barrier. A gentle yet effective cleanser keeps skin looking its best. Never over cleanse your skin.

4. Next lightly apply CP Serum to the face to help repair the skin's protective barrier and antioxidant defenses. In clinical studies at the University of California, SRCPs were able to stimulate skin-barrier repair within 24 to 48 hours.

5. Finish with a light application of Emu Oil-S to help the skin retain a healthy glow.

Chapter 9

SRCP Products for Improving Health of Extra-Sensitive Skin
BioHeal and CP Serum for "At Risk" Skin

> *"When they check for skin sores in the nursing home, the nurses, physicians, and technicians for blood-drawing come in and everyone is nervous. If you have a skin sore, they just slap an expensive bandage on it, which does nothing."*
> — *Comment from a Client in California*

This quote from an elderly client demonstrates an unfortunate reality in the United States: the fact that prevention is not emphasized in our health-care system. Skin care in hospitals and nursing homes often fails to maintain patients' basic skin health. Medicare pays for complicated bandages; therefore, the focus is on selling expensive bandages to cover sores, and there is little interest in low-cost preventative measures (aka, Looting the U.S. Treasury).

In addition to the elderly, people with the following conditions often suffer from extra-sensitive skin:

— Eczema
— Psoriasis
— Very dry skin
— Sjorgren's Syndrome, an autoimmune disease with symptoms of dry and cracking skin
— Thermal or radiation burns
— After chemotherapy treatments
— Skin allergies to materials such as nickel, poison ivy, and poison oak
— Contact dermatitis
— An immune-compromised status (such as HIV or AIDS)

Skin Damaging Conditions and Effects of SRCP Products

Condition Producing Skin Damage	Defect Involved
Diabetes	Inadequate protein synthesis
HIV-Aids Condition	Insufficient immune cells for skin repair
Eczema / Dry Skin / Sjorgen's Syndrome	Damaged skin barrier causes excessive water loss
Contact Dermatitis	Damaged skin barrier allows entry of irritants
Thermal & Radiation Burns	"Zone-of-stasis" around injury blocks blood vessel growth and wound repair
Post - Chemotherapy	Lack of sufficient immune cells for skin repair
Skin Allergies	Antigens cause free radicals that produce an inflamed state
Psoriasis	Abnormal production of skin cells that leads to skin barrier damage

COMPLICATIONS CAUSED BY DAMAGE TO SKIN BARRIER

Skin barrier damage can be rapidly healed at an early stage of breakdown

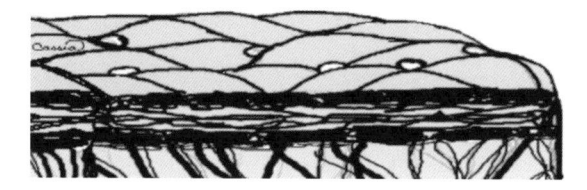

....

IF NOT

Damage to the skin barrier may cause the following:

Irritants may enter causing eczema, skin allergies, and dermatitis

Viruses, fungi, bacteria may enter causing infection

May start skin ulcers (diabetic, bedsores, venous stasis)

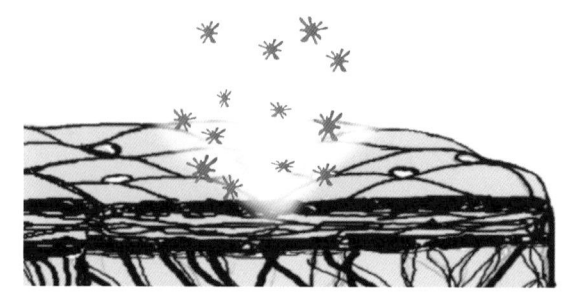

Figure 9.1 © Loren Pickart PhD

BioHeal and CP Serum Can Help

For those with extra-sensitive skin, using SRCP products helps maintain skin health and prevent skin problems. As anyone who suffers from extra-sensitive skin knows, prevention is a much more appealing course of action than healing an open wound once it occurs.

Besides the obvious unpleasantness of an open wound, there is another reason why preventative skin care is important. Healthy skin has a strong resistance to irritants and microorganisms, but once damaged, it is prone to infections, irritants, and allergic reactions. The result is direct damage to the skin itself, an inhibition of the normal skin-repair process, the chronic generation of free radicals in the damaged area, or a combination of the three.

For individuals with limited mobility (such as people in wheelchairs), skin health is a constant concern. Chronic rubbing and pressure on skin areas frequently causes irritation, bedsores, and skin ulcers. Rapid healing of these conditions is vital to avoid the development of serious complications.

I recommend two Skin Biology products in particular to those with extra-sensitive skin: BioHeal and CP Serum. BioHeal is a gentle, safe mineral cream containing protective lipids that helps the body heal damaged skin. It is safer than cortisone and corticosteroids. CP Serum is a mild water-based liquid SRCP that is easy to spread on the skin. Other recommended Skin Biology products for extra-sensitive skin include Gentle Clean (bar or liquid) and Emu Oil-S. In this chapter, you will discover how to effectively treat extra-sensitive and various types of damaged skin with these products.

A word of caution: BioHeal, CP Serum, and other Skin Biology products are designed to improve skin health, but are not substitutes for regular medical care by a qualified health-care professional. They should not be used on broken skin or large, deep wounds. If skin problems persist or worsen, consult a physician.

Photographs at left: Example of healing "at-risk" skin. In the top photo, the patient has two open skin ulcers visible in the left, top and bottom of the photo (A). On the right, there are reddish fissures developing into skin ulcers (B). In the bottom photo, the application of SRCPs to the periphery of the skin ulcers has healed the fissured skin (B) while the open ulcers still remain. It is in the early stages of skin breakdown that skin still can be quickly healed.

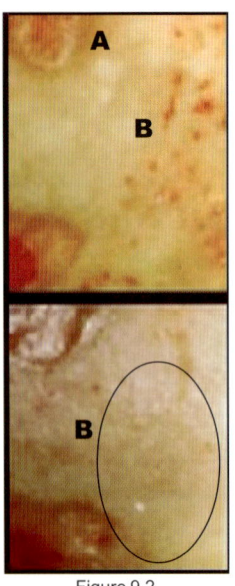

Figure 9.2

BioHeal helps rebuild the protective acid mantle of the skin that many soaps and cleansers strip away (in addition to rebuilding the underlying skin barrier). The acid mantle is the combination of sebum (oils) and perspiration on the skin's surface that protects the skin and renders it less vulnerable to damage and attack by environmental factors, such as sun and wind, and less prone to dehydration. The mantle also has strong antioxidant properties. Sebum is naturally white, but air oxidation turns it black (this is why "whitehead comedos" turn into "blackhead comedos").

Normal skin is somewhat acidic, falling into the pH range of 4.2 to 5.6. This acidity inhibits the growth of foreign bacteria and fungi and the skin remains healthier. Many cleansers and other skin-care products are alkaline (often having a pH of 9 to 10), which can strip off protective oils and exacerbate acne, allergies, and other skin problems.

BioHeal is designed to adjust the skin's pH level into the acidic range. The product contains high levels of lipids such as squalane, cetyl alcohol, glyceryl stearate, and stearic acid that resemble the fats of the acid mantle. Squalane/squalene are the skin's most important protective lipids, but decline as we age (from levels of up to 15 percent in teenagers' skin to less than 5 percent in adults over age 60), resulting in dryer skin. BioHeal also contains allantoin, aloe, Vitamin E, and retinol to aid the mantle's protective antioxidant properties.

Extra-sensitive skin carries a special danger of infection. Immune cells in the skin naturally produce hydrogen peroxide to fight bacteria. Many Skin Biology clients report good results by pre-washing the skin with 3 percent hydrogen peroxide for sterilization and blotting it reasonably dry before applying BioHeal. Some clinicians recommend against the use of hydrogen peroxide on damaged skin because they say it increases skin damage. In contrast, my review of medical literature has found many reports of improved skin healing after washes of hydrogen peroxide at low concentrations (1 to 10 percent). However, skin damage is occasionally observed at higher concentrations of hydrogen peroxide. So any use of hydrogen peroxide on damaged skin should be with concentrations of 1 to 3 percent and no higher.

It Worked for Her!

To understand the dramatic benefits SRCPs have on extra-sensitive and damaged skin, consider the story of Joy Dawson (adapted from the Witchita Eagle newspaper), a 75-year-old middle-school substitute teacher who suffered from eczema, a painful skin inflammation, on her index fingers and thumbs. After reading an article in the Witchita Eagle about non-surgical ways to reduce wrinkles, Joy tried CP Serum on her hands. She had previously tried lotions and salves from her dermatologist, as well as alternative medicine, without success, and was wearing gloves to bed at night at the suggestion of her son, who is a doctor.

Joy's hands were so affected that "there would be cracks and splits, and they'd be bleeding." The newspaper article told how studies have shown that skin treated with copper peptides has less pigmentation, reduced wrinkling, and holds more moisture. The article also mentioned that such creams were originally developed for burn victims and diabetics whose wounds wouldn't heal. Since Joy also suffers from type 2 diabetes, she didn't have to think long about trying CP Serum, which she ordered over the Internet. Within a few weeks, the eczema and cracking skin vanished. Her skin was once again healthy. Joy was very happy with the results!

Treating Eczema

As Joy discovered, eczema responds well to SRCPs. Eczema, a general term for "inflammation of the skin," is a common skin disorder. Usually it is caused by a combination of factors, including a slow skin-repair mechanism, the skin being exposed to many irritants, and the skin being too alkaline. When the skin doesn't have enough acid, a loosening of the outer protective proteins occurs, allowing irritants to pass through. Many clients have found relief from eczema by applying a light coating of BioHeal or CP Serum to the affected area daily, as the following letter shows.

"Dear Sirs:

Thanks for letting me try your BioHeal skin cream on my hand…The area of eczema on my right hand was about 2" long and 1.5" wide, very inflamed, sore, and continuing to spread. The problem started in October 1992 and I had given up hoping for a recovery—all the ointments I had been using allowed, at best, a temporary relief of the itching and burning. These ointments included a 1 percent and a 0.5 percent cortisone cream, a steroid cream prescribed by a doctor, and a coal tar from a health shop. Every time the hand started to look or feel a little better, the eczema would flare up again and I would be back to square one. Conditions that aggravated the eczema included chlorine in our swimming pool, bleach, and perfumed hand creams. I do not know how or why it started in the first place…

Within the first few days of using your cream, I noticed the inflammation was reduced and the eczema had stopped spreading. About two weeks later, the cracks were healing well and the area was no longer tender. Now, three weeks later, there are just a few little scars that are quickly disappearing.

I wish you the best success with the cream. I really thought my problem was here to stay, so thanks again."
-Z.S., London, U.K.

Treating Very Dry Skin

As we age, there is a tendency to develop a drier, less oily skin which is prone to cracks and fissures that may become irritated, inflamed, and itchy. The condition is worse in areas with relatively few oil glands, such as the arms, legs, and trunk. Dry skin occurs more often during the fall and winter because of low humidity combined with frequent bathing. Some dermatologists feel dry skin has worsened in recent decades because people take more baths and showers today. In the past, most people took only one or two baths per year, and the skin had a chance to replace its natural skin oils between baths.

Conventional oil/water moisturizers can temporarily relieve very dry skin, but do not address the fundamental problem and can worsen the condition with time by weakening the skin's outer protective proteins. Biological healing oils, such as Emu Oil-S and Squalane, are the best moisturizers for very dry skin.

Sjorgren's Syndrome

Clients with Sjorgren's Syndrome often prefer TriReduction with Retinol. This product alleviates the dry skin and also helps heal old scars resulting from the syndrome. The following is a letter from such a client:

"I have Sjorgren's Syndrome and Lupus causing severe problems with very dry skin. I am prone to 'cracks' in my fingers due to Raynaud's, and 'burns' in other areas of my skin, including my face. I have used many expensive products trying to help the situation, with minimal results…I have never written about a product before, but the improvement has been so significant…I have been using Protect & Restore and BioHeal for about one month. Since using these creams, my skin is greatly improved with better texture and is significantly less dry. I was afraid to try anything on the burned areas of my face, but went ahead when I saw the improvement in other areas. The burns healed within days. More impressive, the unsightly scars from the steroids have been replaced with healthy skin. I have not had further problems of that type. In the past two weeks, I have received numerous compliments on my skin."–L.A., California

Treating Diabetic Skin Problems

The complications associated with diabetes lead to skin that is dry, tends to crack, and is slow to heal. Rapid repair of broken and cracked skin, before an infection sets in, is very important. Leg and foot sores are the leading cause of amputations associated with broken skin that becomes infected. Many clients who have diabetes and use BioHeal tell us that a daily application of the product to damaged skin usually leads to a quick improvement in skin health.

Treating Skin After Burns, Radiation Treatment, and Chemotherapy

Burns from thermal injuries, radiation treatment, and chemotherapy heal very slowly. After the burn, a "zone-of-stasis" often develops around the burned tissue, and this may turn into an oozing sore or skin ulcer. Under these circumstances, the body does not receive the proper signals to heal the skin. This can result in scarring and permanently damaged skin. Chemotherapy also slows skin repair and increases the development of sores.

For skin that has been damaged in any of these ways, I recommend the use of BioHeal beginning after the burn has scabbed over (about a week post-burn) or treatment has finished. Use a light coating of BioHeal every day in the morning and evening as needed.

"A patient of mine had a chronic sore for four months on her chest after surgery and radiation therapy for breast cancer. Nothing seemed to heal the sore so I tried the BioHeal around the periphery of the sore and it healed over in about three weeks. I had her continue to use the cream on the skin area for another two weeks and the healing has been complete."
- J.D., New York

Treating Allergies

Approximately 25 percent of people are allergic to nickel, and many more are sensitive to plants such as poison ivy and poison oak. BioHeal works well in these situations and is much safer than cortisone and other corticosteroids. Corticosteroids (including cortisone) stop the inflammation but produce damaged and thinned skin (often 50 percent thinner) by inhibiting the natural skin-repair process. Overuse of corticosteroids can promote diabetic conditions, thymus involution, immune suppression, the spread of cancers, bone damage, and cataracts.

In one study, BioHeal both accelerated the recovery of skin after injury and had an anti-inflammatory action on the skin of nickel-allergic subjects who were exposed to nickel salts. (See references in Chapter 16). Many of our clients have also reported rapid healing of insect bites after using BioHeal.

Because allergies are so diverse, it is recommended that you first try BioHeal on a small skin area. If this seems OK, apply a light coating once or twice daily until the allergy is resolved.

"Dear Skin Bio,
I am writing to tell you that your product BioHeal® took away my poison ivy. I have a history of problems with poison ivy since 1975. It is always treated in the same way, first soaps, then cortisone creams in increasing strength. This does not work. It keeps spreading and getting worse. I develop an allergenic reaction to it and end up on prednisone. The prednisone is very hard to take. Last summer I needed to be on the medication for three weeks and suffered through some difficult side effects.

I can't stay away from gardening. I got it about two weeks ago on my hands. It was suggested that I try some Protect and Restore®. I did and it took away the itch immediately and the blisters that were developing never did [develop]. Thank you! I only hope that others that suffer from poison ivy can know about Protect and Restore® and what it can do for them."
-R.W., Minnesota

Treating Contact Dermatitis

Contact dermatitis is an inflammation of the skin caused by direct contact with an irritating substance. This condition is caused by a breakdown of the skin barrier that normally resists irritants and exposure to irritants. Contact dermatitis often occurs after hair-removal methods that increase invasion by bacteria and viruses, such as shaving, waxing, and electrolysis. It is interesting to note that most warts occur in frequently shaved areas, including the legs of women and the beard area in men. The more rapidly affected skin is healed, the better the skin's protection against viruses and bacteria.

Contact dermatitis can also be caused by nail-polish removers containing acetone or acetonitrile, which act to extract skin fats and damage the skin on the fingers and cuticle of the nails. This can produce hangnails, skin flaking and increased allergies.

If you suffer from contact dermatitis, applying BioHeal to the affected area will help accelerate healing, as the following letter shows.

"In researching contact dermatitis around the eyes, this was the ONLY site on the Web describing the condition. I ordered some CP Serum (already had Squalane) and Emu Oil-S. I have a cabinet full of oils that I purchased to get rid of this condition. Only the CP Serum and Emu Oil-S or Squalane helped heal it. I wasn't even able to wear makeup…I can now use Super CP and all my makeup. My eyes are looking great."-J.B.

AIDS and Skin Health

Persons with AIDS and HIV face constant difficulties in maintaining dermal health. Small abrasions and cuts heal very slowly because of the depressed immune function. Skin infections are a constant threat that can rapidly become annoying exudative lesions and mycotic infections. The SRCPs in products such as BioHeal and CP Serum have been shown to restore normal skin repair and hair growth in animals made immunosuppressed by pretreatment with cortisone or chemotherapeutic drugs (See references in Chapter 16). However, neither product has been approved by the FDA for use on open wounds or skin ulcers.

"Your copper blue cream really helps with my multiple skin annoyances associated with living with HIV for 14 years and AIDS now for 5 years. BioHeal is wonderful for my face to keep down the usually exudative type mycotic lesions and infectious irritations which are gone now after the Bioheal cream."
- V.F., California

Treating Psoriasis

Five million people in the United States suffer from psoriasis, a skin condition that produces an inflamed, itchy, thickened, and cracked skin. Many Skin Biology clients with psoriasis have reported that applying BioHeal to the affected area daily alleviates the problems associated with mild psoriasis outbreaks. In 1996, Professor DiJun Rong of Shanghai Medical University wrote Skin Biology a letter saying that in psoriasis patients treated with BioHeal, the thickness of the lesions was thinned, itching was reduced, and the quality of the skin improved. Here's another letter describing the positive effect SRCPs have on psoriasis.

"Hello there, Dr. Pickart!
...I wanted to let you know that P&R [Protect & Restore, another SRCP product] has virtually eliminated my mother's psoriasis. It is truly amazing—she had a large patch on her right forearm that was constantly irritated from rubbing against the armrest of her wheelchair, and nothing was helping, so I gave her a tube...It showed immediate improvement, so when she finished one tube, and the psoriasis was diminished by about 50 percent, we got her another tube right away. Once that one was finished, there was just a light trace left, and we ordered a 4-ounce tube. She's barely gotten started on that one, and it's practically gone!...She will never be without your product again!"
- D.H., Texas

SRCPs Plus Emu Oil-S

An even better response can be obtained by those using SRCPs to treat eczema, psoriasis, and other skin conditions when the application of BioHeal or CP Serum is followed with Emu Oil-S. The fatty acid composition of human skin oil and emu oil are very similar. This may be the reason for the positive actions of emu oil on human skin[1].

Numerous studies have shown the effectiveness of emu oil. A study by Lopez and colleagues (1999) found strong anti-inflammatory effects of topically applied emu oil after skin was exposed to a very strong irritant.[2] Politis and Dmytrowich (1998) found that if emu oil was applied two days after injury, it aided the healing process. Researchers at the University of Texas Medical School found emu oil at up to 100 percent concentration in lotions to be non-allergenic, non-comedogenic, bacteriostatic, and to have low irritation potential.[3] Throughout history, emu oil has been used to help alleviate the discomfort of skin conditions such as arthritis, shingles, eczema, psoriasis, and other inflammatory conditions. (References in Chapter 20).

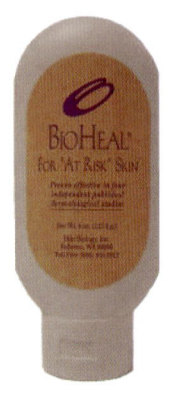

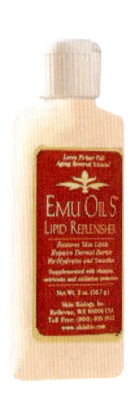

> *"I don't want baby skin,
> I want the skin of a babe."*
> — *Los Angeles Client*

Chapter 10

Keeping Your Skin Young & Beautiful

What is beautiful skin? In every culture, the most coveted skin is that of a young person between the ages of 10 and 20. The impact of having clear, blemish-free skin on other people is powerful; psychological studies of 170 human cultures have found this to be the No. 1 factor in interpersonal attraction.

Beyond the musings of poets, the characteristics of what is considered beautiful skin generally include:

— A firm, elastic tone
— Smooth and free of defects
— Often has some lingering traces of "baby fat"
— A reddish tint (regardless of skin color) from profuse blood circulation
— Usually is somewhat suntanned
— Free of skin breaks and cracks
— A clear, vivid look

Biologically, these characteristics translate into skin with the following:
- A healthy acid mantle and strong protein/lipid skin barrier
- A rapid turnover of skin cells
- Collagen and elastin fibers in excellent repair
- A constantly renewed blood circulation, ensuring an adequate flow of nutrients to the skin
- Ample levels of water-holding proteoglycans and glycosaminoglycans
- The ability to heal itself rapidly after injury
- High antioxidant levels and superoxide dismutase activity
- Adequate but not excessive natural skin oils
- A high level of subcutaneous fat cells

With the proper skin-care regimen, beautiful skin is within your grasp. In this chapter, you will learn about many of the components of healthy skin and what you can do to keep your skin young and beautiful.

> *"The skin of a delicate woman is an example of softness and smoothness united."*
> — Uvedale Price

The Protective Skin Barrier

Research shows that healthy skin has a strong resistance to damage and irritation. The part of your skin that protects you from the elements is known as the protective skin barrier. This barrier consists of three components: 1) the acid mantle, 2) the hard outer skin proteins tightly glued together by lipids and 3) the underlying supply of immune cells that guard against viruses and bacteria.

When the barrier function is compromised, the skin is left vulnerable and damage may result. This damage might include warts, moles, bacterial and viral infections, allergic responses, dry skin, inhibited skin repair, more rapid aging, blotches or rashes. As an example, consider someone who is sensitive to wool clothing. If the person has a healthy skin barrier, the wool never reaches the reactive immune cells (Langerhans cells) in the skin. But imagine that the person wearing wool is a soldier in a wet, muddy environment. This combination of conditions puts the soldier at risk for protective barrier damage. Since a damaged skin barrier loses water rapidly, the skin becomes dry, flaky, cracked, inflamed and prone to infection.

Maintaining the Skin Barrier

One way to preserve your protective skin barrier is to maintain a healthy acid mantle. The acid mantle is a combination of sebum (oily fats) and perspiration that is constantly secreted to cover the skin's surface. Normal skin pH is somewhat acidic in the range of 4.2 to 5.6. It varies from one part of the body to another and, in general, the pH of a man's skin is lower (more acidic) than that of a woman's.

The acid mantle benefits your skin in the following ways.

The mantle as antioxidant. An antioxidant is a chemical that prevents the oxidation of other chemicals and in some cases helps the body fight infection. In the acid mantle, the lipids are sacrificially oxidized to protect the underlying skin from excessive oxidation. This is why "whiteheads," which are un-oxidized sebum in pores, turn into "blackheads."

The mantle as water repellent. The fats in the acid mantle repel water from the skin much as the oil on a duck's feathers repels water. This keeps water from loosening and damaging the skin's outer layers of hard protective proteins and lipids and renders the skin less vulnerable to damage and attack by environmental factors, such as sun and wind, and less prone to dehydration.

The mantle as bacterial inhibitor. The acid pH of the mantle inhibits bacterial growth on the skin, especially the growth of foreign pathogenic bacteria and fungi. As a result, the skin remains healthier and has fewer blemishes.

The mantle protects the skin barrier. The skin barrier is hard keratin proteins glued together by lipids. Keratin must be kept at an acid pH to keep the protective proteins tightly bound together and to maintain its hardness. More alkaline pHs weaken the lipid glue and soften and loosen the fibers of keratin. This creates gaps in the barrier that allows allergens, irritants, bacteria and viruses to penetrate into the skin. Acne, skin allergies and other skin problems become more severe when the skin becomes more alkaline.

Protecting Your Delicate Skin

Your skin is delicate, and as such needs to be cared for with a delicate hand. The following methods effectively minimize damage to the skin.

> *A few hundred years ago, Marie Antoinette shocked the French court by bathing at least weekly — the French Aristocracy stuck to their twice yearly baths.*

1. Cleanse your face and hands, and take baths and showers only as needed (no more than once a day). Too much cleansing removes the skin's natural oil layer, which increases evaporation of the skin's moisture. The skin's oils are necessary to retain water. It is this naturally retained water that increases the skin's suppleness and softness. Showers are better for your skin than baths because they soak the skin less and are less drying. If you have skin irritations or dry skin, use lukewarm water; hot water is more drying to the skin. Limit your time to 15 minutes or less in the bath or shower. Use a minimum amount of soap. Long, hot baths, although wonderfully relaxing, should be limited to once or twice a week.

Take care of your skin after cleansing. When toweling, gently rub the skin. Blot or pat the skin dry so there is still some moisture left on it. Apply a biological healing oil, such as Emu Oil-S, Squalane, or squalane/octyl-palmitate, after bathing.

2. Use a mild soap. Keeping your skin's pH at the proper level means choosing your soap carefully. Since each pH unit has a 10-fold difference in alkalinity, soap with a pH of 10.5 has 10 times the alkalinity of soap with a pH of 9.5. Even "mild" soaps are often quite alkaline (with a pH of 9.5 to 11) and can damage the skin by stripping away the acid mantle. Most soaps also contain a high level of synthetic detergents, which loosen the protective wall of keratin proteins and lipids. Irritated and eczematous skin tends to have a more alkaline pH, and washing with soap can increase this alkaline state and make the skin even more vulnerable to irritation and infection.

Strong soaps remove our naturally occurring skin bacteria that protects us from the establishment of harmful, disease-causing bacteria. Deodorant soaps are harsh and are not recommended. Limit the use of soap to areas that develop an odor, such as the armpits, genital area, and feet. Make sure all the soap is rinsed from your skin after washing or before you leave the tub or shower.

Skin Biology has developed a cleanser for sensitive and damaged skin called Gentle Clean that was originally developed for the fragile skin of cancer patients after chemotherapy or radiation treatments. The cleanser comes as a clear, translucent bar or liquid and contains no harsh detergents, caustics or "flash" foaming agents. The pH is 7.5, far below the alkalinity of other soaps. Nurses and physicians report that Gentle Clean works well on sensitive and fragile skin such as that which occurs with eczema, psoriasis, diabetes, in the bedridden and after cancer therapy. Fragile skin can literally be dissolved by strong soaps.

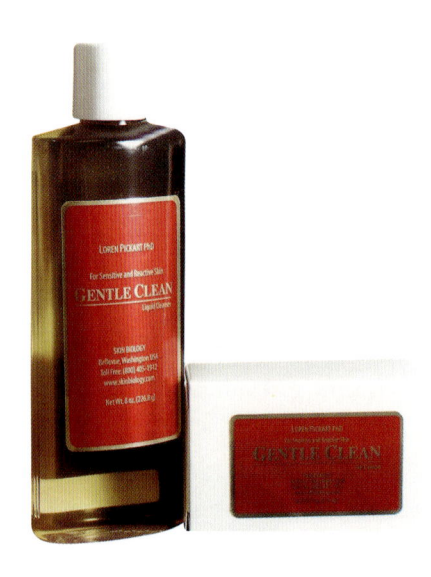

3. Saunas, hot tubs and steam baths are good alternatives to bathing and showering and cleanse the skin without soap. Users generally have very beautiful skin.

The high heat generated by saunas, hot tubs and steam baths has an almost magical effect on the body. It has been found to improve blood flow, lower blood pressure, kill disease organisms and inhibit cancer growth. Some gerontologists have suggested that high heat may increase free-radical production in the body. However, the maximum life span of humans in warm areas of the world is similar to that in cold areas. Many cold-blooded reptiles are short-lived, while birds such as crows, with a temperature of 105 to 110 degrees F, can live for more than 90 years.

Saunas, hot tubs and steam baths soften pore-clogging oils and waxes, allowing for normal pore function and the removal of pore-clogging waxes. The skin is a major excretory organ for wastes, and the heat-induced perspiration cleans the accumulated residue of dead cells, rancid oils, bacteria and perspiration wastes.

Some caution is necessary when starting sauna, hot tub and/or steam-bath use. Let your body adapt over several weeks before increasing the temperature of the unit and the time you spend in it. Do not eat for two hours before heating your body. You should not raise your body temperature above about 105 degrees F, even after becoming acclimated. After using a sauna, hot tub or steam bath, let your body cool down slowly, for the same reason as you would after vigorous exercise—to allow your vascular system to readjust to normal function.

Pregnant women should exercise special caution when using saunas, hot tubs and steam baths, but can benefit greatly from their use. A study of Finnish women, of whom 98.5 percent use saunas while pregnant, found common birth defects to be among the lowest of any country in the world[1].

Never use a sauna, hot tub or steam bath if you have been drinking alcohol. Alcohol coupled with the heat can cause extreme vasodilation, and blood pressure can drop to a point where you become unconscious. Inebriated hot-tubbers have been found after several days of slow cooking in the tub.

4. Avoid astringents and toners, which are drying to the skin. They make the face look very clean and smooth by stripping away the top layer of oil and briefly tightening the skin. However, the skin responds by increasing oil production.

5. Many skin researchers consider pure squalane from olive oil to be the best sexual lubricant. It is not sold by skincare companies because of squalane's relatively high wholesale cost.

6. Filling your home with plants is one of the best ways of adding humidity to the air and reducing dry skin. Alternately, a water humidifier will keep indoor air at healthy humidity levels.

Increasing Skin Cell Turnover

Another way to preserve the protective skin barrier is to keep a constant flow of cells moving outward in the skin to supply new proteins and lipids to replace the older, outer skin layers. For those over age 30, the regular use of SRCPs and the skin's natural hydroxy acids will speed skin-cell turnover. For skin maintenance, weekly use mild or moderate strength SRCPs 3 to 4 times and an exfoliating agent such as 7 to 10 percent lactic acid or 1 to 2 percent salicylic acid (three times should suffice). Another option is to also use retinoic acid two to three times a week.

Manual exfoliation also works well. Methods of manual exfoliation include using a skin brush, a pumice stone or a buffer. Some of our clients abrade with a spot scraper to "flake-off" damage. Microdermabrasion and needling can also prove successful in removing damaged skin.

Special Needs of the Eyelids

The eyelids, the thinnest skin on the body, require special attention. Before applying eye cosmetics, first apply a light protective layer of CP Serum, Super CP Serum, or Protect & Restore. These products provide a protective coating with antioxidant protection. Then use a minimum amount of eye shadow, eye liner, and mascara. Remove eye makeup with either Emu Oil-S for Skin or pure Squalane. Most cosmetic makeup removers are very harsh and damaging to delicate skin.

Controlling Oily Skin, Sebum, Blackheads and Acne

Oily skin with excessive sebum production can harden and form comedos that block pores. Comedos start as whiteheads, but then air oxidation darkens the sebum to form blackheads. The bacteria in the blocked pores multiplies, producing the irritation that becomes acne.

If you have blackheads, a good treatment option is pore-cleansing strips. These are "paste-on" strips coated with an adhesive glue that bonds to the blackhead. The strip is applied to skin, allowed to dry, and then pulled off along with the blackhead. But do not overuse these to the point of skin irritation.

Reducing Pore Size

As we age, our skin becomes thinner and pores become more prominent. Contrary to what magazine advertisements tell you, oil-removing solutions do not reduce pore size, but rather cause the skin to produce more oil and larger pores to compensate for the removed oil.

In contrast, both retinoic acid and lactic acid reduce oil production and pore size. Increasing your rate of skin renewal also reduces pore size, since the firmer and thicker skin helps squeeze the pore downward and inward. Skin renewal serums and creams that increase collagen, elastin, proteoglycans and the amount of subcutaneous fat (the very thin layer under the skin) both firm the skin and increase its thickness. Our clients often tell us that Super CP Serum works well for this purpose.

Protecting Your Hands

There are specific things you can do to protect the skin of your hands. One of these is wearing vinyl gloves whenever you come in contact with household chemicals and other harsh elements. Wear the gloves when folding laundry, peeling vegetables or handling citrus fruits or tomatoes. Purchase four or five pair and keep them in the kitchen, bathroom, nursery and laundry areas. Have other pairs for non-wet housework and gardening. Avoid latex gloves, since many people are sensitive to them. Dry out the gloves between cleaning jobs. When outdoors in cool weather, wear unlined leather gloves to protect against dry and chapped skin. It will also benefit your hands if you are careful with them when washing dishes or clothes. Avoid hand-washing items if you can, and if you must, keep your hands out of the soapy water as much as possible. Using an automatic dishwasher will protect your hands and also effectively sterilize your dishes. Remove rings whenever washing or working with your hands. When you wash your hands, use lukewarm water and very little soap.

Aerobic Exercise Improves Skin Health

Aerobic exercise markedly improves skin quality and overall body health. Mail carriers, who spend their days walking, have the longest lifespan of any occupational group in the United States. Many people who live to advanced ages have a life filled with long walks. Physical ability decreases less with age than commonly believed; the body "wears out" faster from a lack of use than overuse.

The benefits of aerobic exercise are too numerous to list. Exercise increases the blood capillary density in the skin and improves the nutrition of skin cells. It increases overall body metabolism and retards many of the effects of aging. In one study, healthy men in their 50's who exercised vigorously displayed a tissue oxygen uptake capacity and cardiovascular function that was 20 to 30 percent higher than sedentary young men.[2]

Ideally, you should get between three and five hours of vigorous aerobic exercise a week. Researchers have found that moderate exercise is as healthful as stressful exercise. The best forms of exercise are fun and reduce your stress level. Do what makes you happy and feel good. Golf, hiking, walking, hunting, fishing and even gardening are all good options.

Once you establish an exercise routine that works for you, keep it up! Unless you are an elite athlete, if you start skipping workouts, the ability of your muscles to produce aerobic energy will rapidly decrease, dropping by 50 percent in just one week. After five to 12 days, your capillary density will decrease by 10 to 20 percent and the capacity of your heart to pump blood will diminish. Two months of inactivity will wipe out about 90 percent of the conditioning gained through exercise.[3]

Biological Skin Oils vs. Cosmetic Moisturizers

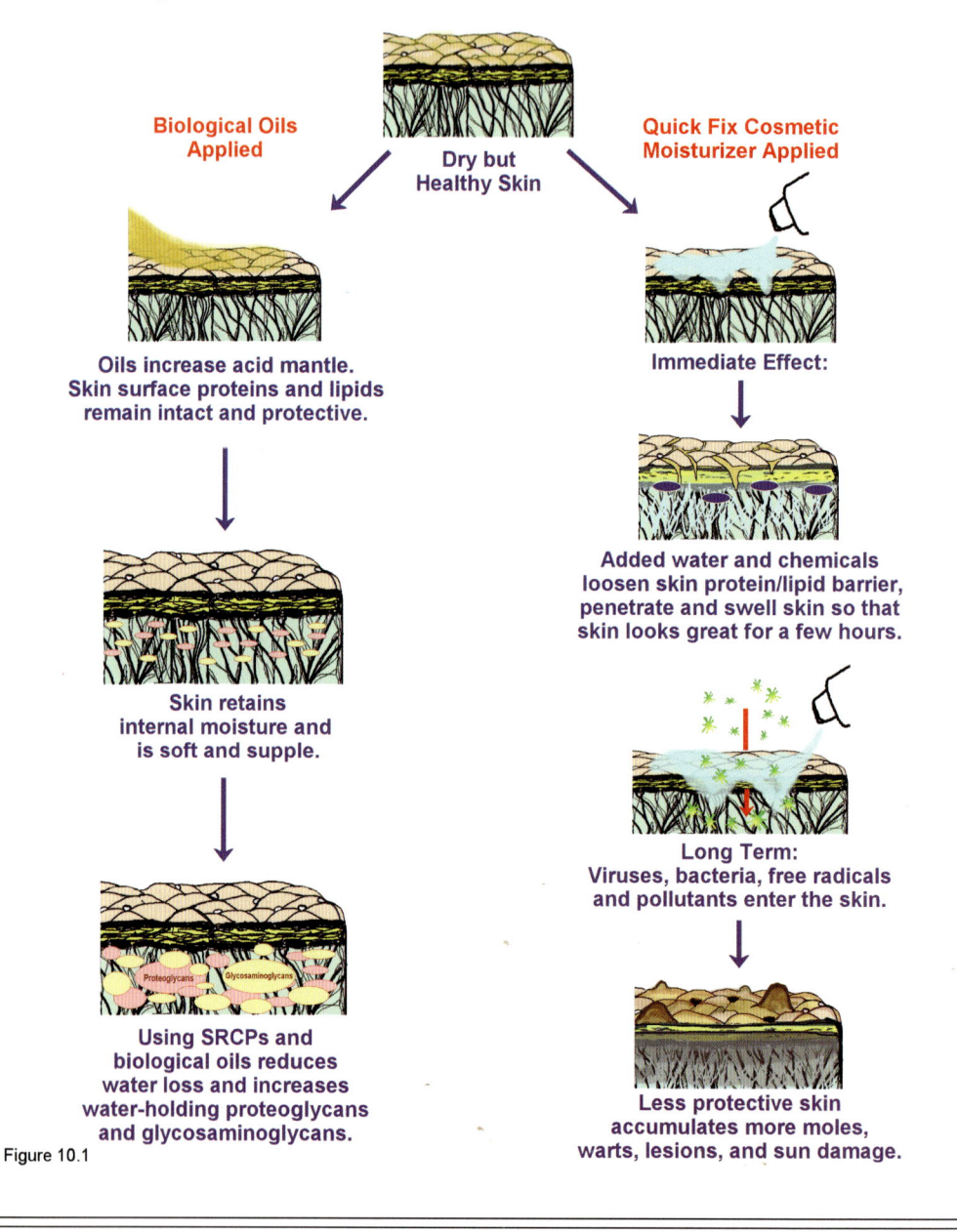

Dry but Healthy Skin

Biological Oils Applied

Oils increase acid mantle. Skin surface proteins and lipids remain intact and protective.

Skin retains internal moisture and is soft and supple.

Using SRCPs and biological oils reduces water loss and increases water-holding proteoglycans and glycosaminoglycans.

Quick Fix Cosmetic Moisturizer Applied

Immediate Effect:

Added water and chemicals loosen skin protein/lipid barrier, penetrate and swell skin so that skin looks great for a few hours.

Long Term: Viruses, bacteria, free radicals and pollutants enter the skin.

Less protective skin accumulates more moles, warts, lesions, and sun damage.

Figure 10.1

Treating Dry Skin with Biological Healing Oils

Dry skin is caused by two problems: 1) Damage to the skin's protective barrier, which produces excessive water loss through the skin, and 2) a reduction in the concentrations of the skin's water-holding sugars and proteins, the proteoglycans and glycosaminoglycans (GAGs). Treating dry skin with a biological healing oil, such as emu oil or squalane, can help. Biological healing oils are superior to the moisturizers made by cosmetics companies, which loosen the skin's protective barrier and can actually damage the skin.

For thousands of years, our ancestors used biological healing oils to improve the health of their skin. But around 1920, the cosmetic industry began advertising the idea that these oils are bad for the skin and promoting the use of oil/water/detergent mixtures instead. This was similar to campaigns to stop women from breastfeeding their babies so that synthetic infant formulas could be sold. In reality, nothing could be further from the truth. The next two sections describe the benefits of emu oil and squalane on the skin.

> *"Thou anointest my head with oil...*
> *My cup runneth over."*
> *– 23rd Psalm of King David*

> *"The great hearted Odysseus was home at last.*
> *The maid Eurynome bathed him,*
> *rubbed him down with oil,*
> *and drew around him a royal cape..."*
> *– Homer 800 B.C.*

Emu Oil

Australian aborigines discovered the benefits of emu oil thousands of years ago. The fatty acid composition of human skin oil and emu oil is similar. In both oils, monounsaturated oleic acid is the most prevalent element, then palmitic acid, followed by linoleic acid (an essential fatty acid).

One of emu oil's many benefits is that it is an excellent natural oil for lipid replacement and often accelerates skin repair and can be a helpful treatment for dry skin, as well as eczema, burns and psoriasis.

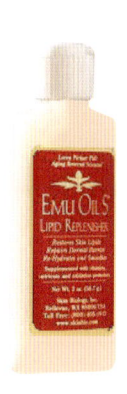

Emu oil has special benefits for damaged skin. A study at Texas Tech reported that topically applied emu oil reduces burn pain as effectively as 600 mgs of Ibuprofen taken three times daily. Another study, by Lopez and colleagues, found that emu oil had strong anti-inflammatory effects after skin was exposed to croton oil, a very strong irritant. Twelve hours after applying the emu oil, there was significantly less edema and swelling.[4] Politis and Dmytrowich found that if emu oil is applied two days after an injury, it aids the healing process. However, they also found that when emu oil is applied immediately after an injury, it delays healing.[5] So for skin repair, first use an SRCP product to help start repair, and then later start using the emu oil.

Skin Biology's Emu Oil-S Lipid Replenisher for Skin is a peroxide-free emu oil supplemented with Co-Q10, mixed isomers of natural tocotrienols, lutein, lycopene, and mixed isomers of vitamin E all of which are powerful antioxidants. Skin Biology also makes an emu oil product for the hair, Emu Oil-S Lipid Replenisher for Hair, a peroxide-free emu oil supplemented with similar antioxidants and saw palmetto oil.

The ingredients in Skin Biology's emu oil products were carefully selected. Tocotrienols selectively accumulate in skin and serve to protect it against ultraviolet damage and oxidation. In rats it was found that UV radiation significantly reduced vitamin E concentrations after 29 minutes of UV exposure, but in skin treated with tocotrienols, the vitamin E concentrations were seven to 30 times higher after the radiation.[6] Lutein and lycopene are powerful antioxidants that naturally exist in the human body. CoQ-10 functions in the energy production in the mitochondria of cells. It also serves as a lipid-soluble antioxidant in the skin. Animals fed CoQ-10 have lower cancer rates.

When using emu oil, apply a light coating to your skin or scalp. If your skin feels too oily, lightly wipe off the excess oil with a tissue (enough of the oil will stick to your skin to be effective).

Squalane

Squalane and squalene are two very similar lipids. Together they compose 15 percent of the skin fats in teenagers' skin, but decline to about 5 percent after age 50. This is a major factor in the skin becoming rough, dry, and vulnerable to damage.

For thousands of years, fishermen from Scandinavia, Japan, and the South Pacific have used fish fats rich in squalane/squalene for healing the skin of their faces and hands after irritation by salt water. Squalane from olive oil is mainly used today. Squalane/squalene serves as an antioxidant for cell membranes and within the cell. The compounds have some anti-cancer properties and promote the activity of T and B lymphocytes and macrophages.[7] Mice were protected against the toxicity and injury of radiation when fed a diet supplemented with 2 percent Squalane.[8] The compounds also have some anti-fungal properties and enhance the effects of Amphotericin B (Fungizone) against a variety of candida species.[9]

Regular application of squalane helps to maintain your skin's natural moisture level and produces the appearance of softer, smoother skin. It is absorbed deeply and quickly into the skin and does not leave an oily film. It is especially useful on dry, scaly portions of the body.

Psychological Stress Damages Skin

Psychological stress plays a role in skin aging. A study of medical, dental, and pharmacy students assessed their skin barrier recovery from four weeks before final examinations until four weeks after final exams during spring vacation. There was a noteworthy decline in skin barrier protection and healing during the stressful time of studying for exams. But during spring vacation, skin health recovered. According to the researchers who conducted the study, "The greatest deterioration in barrier function occurred in those subjects who demonstrated the largest increases in perceived psychological stress."[10]

Another study confirmed that psychological stress has a negative effect on the skin. The subjects were female volunteers who underwent a night of sleep deprivation, a three-day exercise regimen, and the psychosocial stress of an interview. The conclusion was clear: "Acute psychosocial stress and sleep deprivation disrupts skin barrier function homeostasis in women."[10]

SRCPs for Luscious Lips

To treat dry, chapped lips, many Skin Biology clients apply TriReduction with Retinol or Emu Oil-S for Skin. Female long-distance runners have reported that TriReduction with Retinol provides protection to lips that are constantly exposed to the elements. Some clients have noted that the SRCPs in TriReduction and the deep moisturization of Emu Oil-S give the lips a "fuller" appearance. Protecting your lips is certainly part of keeping your skin looking young and beautiful.

Methods of Skin Moisturization

Method	How It Works	Time to be Effective	Problems	Recommended
SRCPs	Mimics natural repair, repairs skin barrier, and increases the skin's proteoglycans and GAGs	About 2-3 weeks	None	Protect & Restore and CP Serum
Waxes and Greases	Heavy oils such as petrolatum seal skin surface to water loss	Immediate	May disrupt the skin barrier	No
Biological Oils	Oils such as octyl palmitate and squalane help reduce water loss. Oils similar to human skin oils: Emu Oil-S and Squalane	Immediate	Not as durable as waxes and greases but stimulates skin repair	Calypso's Oil Octyl-palmitate, Squalane, and Emu Oil-S Lipid Replenisher
Retinol in Squalane	Increases natural skin oils	2 weeks	Avoid acne-prone areas	Retinol in Squalane
Quick Fix Cosmetic Moisturizers	Designed to improve the look of skin at cosmetic counters. Mixtures of oils, water, and surface-active chemicals that rapidly swell the skin by rapid water uptake	5 minutes	Acts like irritant to loosen protective skin barrier, skin more susceptible to infection	No

Chapter 11

Improving Hair Growth and Condition with SRCPs

When we are young, the hair on our head is thick, well-pigmented, and fast growing. But the passage of time takes a toll, and our hair begins to thin or vanish, grow more slowly, and turn gray. While the search for methods to restore healthy, younger hair is ancient, the reality is that, even today, in the era of Rogaine® (minoxidil) and Propecia® (finasteride), the therapies that profess to restore hair health give a marginal result at best.

While far from a miracle therapy, research on SRCPs has uncovered an unexpected benefit: they have a positive action on the hair follicle function in humans. More and more, SRCPs are being used to improve hair growth and condition, with promising results.

Why the Big Apple is a Bad Hair Town

The effect of the hair-care industry on hair health has been overwhelmingly negative in the opinion of many people, including Russian Physician George Michael. Dr. Michael immigrated to New York City with his family after the 1917 revolution; later he set up a medical practice. Despite the city's abundance of hair salons and other businesses that cater to hair, Michael was immediately struck by how poor the quality of the women's hair was. He reminisced that, in the Russia of his youth, many women in their 60's and beyond had healthy, well-pigmented, waist-length locks, whereas in New York City the women had difficulty growing their hair longer than six inches. Dr. Michael concluded that it was the excess of dyes, cutting, blow drying, relaxers, and so on that was damaging the women's hair. He went on to become the guru of long-hair care, opening a chain of Long Hair Clinics and working with famous long-haired beauties such as Crystal Gayle. (For more information on Dr. Michael, visit Jennifer Bahney's www.longhairlovers.com).

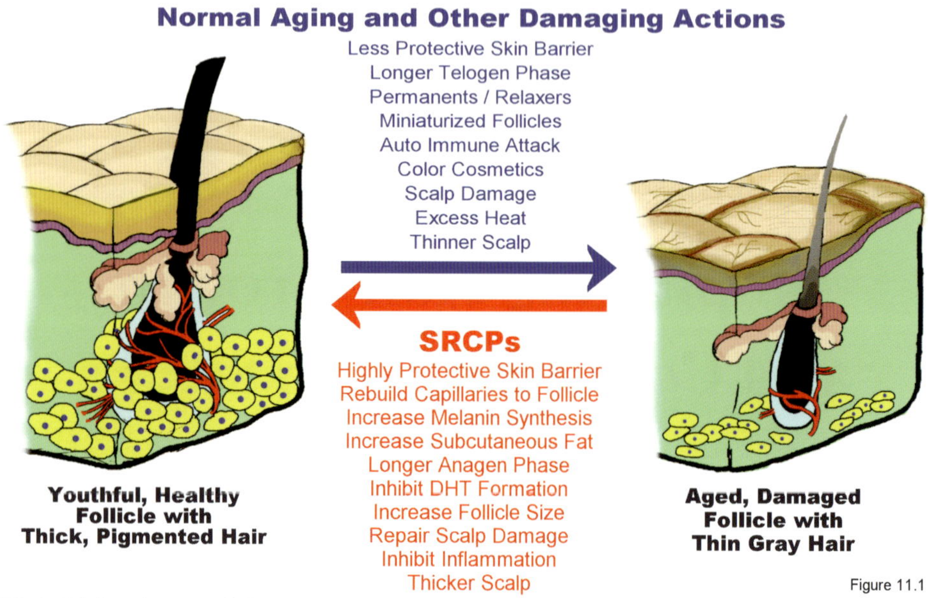

Normal Aging and Other Damaging Actions

Less Protective Skin Barrier
Longer Telogen Phase
Permanents / Relaxers
Miniaturized Follicles
Auto Immune Attack
Color Cosmetics
Scalp Damage
Excess Heat
Thinner Scalp

SRCPs
Highly Protective Skin Barrier
Rebuild Capillaries to Follicle
Increase Melanin Synthesis
Increase Subcutaneous Fat
Longer Anagen Phase
Inhibit DHT Formation
Increase Follicle Size
Repair Scalp Damage
Inhibit Inflammation
Thicker Scalp

Youthful, Healthy Follicle with Thick, Pigmented Hair

Aged, Damaged Follicle with Thin Gray Hair

Figure 11.1

Hair Thinning and Loss

While the cosmetic rigors many women put their hair through undoubtedly have a negative impact on its condition, this is but one of many causes of hair thinning and loss. These causes are more diverse than is generally realized. Most of the scientific theories of hair thinning and loss focus on the metabolic actions of dihydrotestosterone (DHT), but in reality there are many other factors at work. The following is a description of the factors that can inhibit hair growth.

> "One lock of hair falling across the temples has an effect too alluring to be strictly decent."
> —William Hogarth, 1753

DHT and testosterone. The actions of the androgens DHT and testosterone are a major factor in hair growth. These androgens stimulate axillary, pubic, and beard-hair growth (but not the growth of the eyebrows and eyelashes). In the hair follicle, testosterone is enzymatically converted by 5-Alpha Reductase (5-AR) to DHT, which is thought to be a major factor in male pattern baldness (androgenetic alopecia). However, many men with high DHT levels never suffer hair loss. Researchers have concluded that the ultimate factor in hair loss isn't DHT, but damage to the hair follicles. A recent study of 3,000 individuals found no link between baldness and the production of DHT. While DHT plays a key role in hair loss, a final insult of auto-immune damage to the hair follicle may stop hair growth. Some researchers are of the opinion that if follicular health is improved or maintained, it is possible that hair loss can be reversed or minimized.[1]

Miniaturized follicles. At age 15, hair follicles actively produce thick, heavy terminal hair for about three-and-a-half years during the anagen phase, and then shrink for about four months during the dormant telogen phase. As we age, the follicle's anagen phase progressively shortens, while the telogen phase lengthens. The result is a progressive shrinkage of follicle size during the anagen phase, which produces thinner, slower-growing hair. That's why hair conditioners were created: to thicken the hair shaft with fats and proteins and give the hair a fuller, more youthful appearance.[2]

Increase in length of dormant follicle phase. While the increase in the length of the dormant follicle phase is usually attributed to DHT actions, other factors, such as damage caused by excessive heat, coloring agents, and relaxers, may also produce follicle damage that results in less functional follicles.[2]

Inadequate follicle microcirculation. The synthesis of new hair necessitates a very high nutrient flow to the follicle bulb. Morphological studies often observe a markedly diminished capillary blood supply in aged, miniaturized follicles. This alone may be the cause of follicle miniaturization and inadequate hair syntheses.[3]

Inflammation around follicles. Many dysfunctional follicles appear to have an auto-immune inflammation. It has been proposed that this inflammation around the follicle is the final step in the sequence that ultimately produces inactive follicles that are incapable of producing thick, terminal hair.[3]

Decreased subcutaneous fat layer. The layer of fat at the base of the skin, known as subcutaneous adipose tissue or "baby fat", diminishes with age. Researchers have noted the accumulation of this fat around healthy follicles that are vigorously growing hair and a relative lack of it around dormant follicles. They postulate that these fat cells serve a supportive function for the hair follicle. Conditions that inhibit hair growth, such as chemotherapy and starvation, also decrease the subcutaneous fat layer.[3]

Lack of sulfur donors. Hair is composed of 35 percent sulfur-containing amino acids. Only the feathers in birds have a similar level of amino acids. Nutritional sulfur supplements, such as methyl sulfonyl methane (MSM), have long been used to improve the coats of racehorses and are increasingly being used to improve hair health in humans.

Damage from relaxers, excessive heat, coloring agents, and dyes. As previously mentioned, numerous common procedures damage the health of the scalp and hair follicles. Scalp damage from relaxers, permanents, color cosmetics with their organic dyes and metallic salts, and excessive heat from blow dryers and hot oil treatments can literally boil the follicles and also damage the hair shaft's hard outer layers of keratin. When used in combination, these procedures can damage the hair follicles and reduce hair growth. This is often noticeable in women as a decrease or loss of eyebrows and eyelashes around age 40.

Excessive hair cutting. Dr. George Michael emphasized that longer hair is healthier hair. It is possible that the hair follicles thrive from the tension produced by the weight of a heavy hair shaft in the same manner that muscles and bones respond to being exercised.

Additional Causes of Hair Thinning and Loss for Women

Women's hair can also be affected by one or more of the following:

Extreme exercise. In women, severe exercise tends to reduce estrogen and raise testosterone. This can lead to a stopping of the menstrual cycle, brittle bones, and hair thinning or loss. While there are many positive aspects of exercise, there can be too much of a good thing.

Sudden hormone shifts. In women, hair loss can become severe after giving birth to a child or discontinuing the use of oral contraceptives. In these cases, a brief therapy with hair stimulators can usually restore hair to its previous condition.

Reduction of estrogen. Estrogen, the feminizing hormone, can inhibit or counteract the follicle-shrinking effect of androgens. Women have more estrogen circulating in their blood than men. As a result, even women with a genetic predisposition for pattern hair loss are protected from losing their hair. When these women reach menopause, however, their estrogen level may decrease significantly, and the protective effect of the estrogen may be overridden by the DHT message. Then the hair can begin to thin, sometimes rapidly. An estrogen supplementation or DHT blocker may help.

Using SRCPs to Stimulate Hair Growth

One of the many exciting developments in skin research in recent years was the finding that hair follicles are the source of stem cells for the skin. However, long before this discovery linking hair follicles and skin repair, I had observed that, after treating skin wounds with GHK-Cu, there was a profound enlargement of the hair follicles of the skin at the wound edge.

Since then, SRCPs have been proven to:
- Increase hair growth in humans
- Increase hair follicle size in humans
- Improve the "take" of transplanted hair plugs
- Reduce hair loss caused by chemotherapeutic drugs
- Increase the recovery of hair loss caused by chemotherapeutic drugs

An in-depth discussion of the above actions can be found in Chapter 16, The Science Behind SRCPs.

Improving Hair Vitality with SRCPs

> *"Long let me inhale, deeply the odor of your hair, into it plunge the whole of my face, as a thirsty man into the water of a spring, and wave it in my fingers like a scented handkerchief, to shake the memories into the air."*
> — Charles Baudelaire

While recent studies are encouraging, SRCPs are not a miracle cure for hair loss. A more important future use of SRCPs may be as a regular scalp treatment or hair tonic, used once or twice weekly, for the enhancement of hair and scalp health. SRCPs have numerous actions that may improve the hair and scalp. These include:

Reducing DHT formation in hair follicles. 5-alpha reductase (5-AR) exists in two forms: type 1, which functions in hair follicles, and type 2, which acts in prostate tissue. Follicle-damaging DHT is produced in the hair follicles. Propecia (finasteride), a prescription treatment for hair loss in men who have male pattern baldness, inhibits 5-AR throughout the body and improves hair growth. But it works best on the type 2 form and is best suited for controlling prostate enlargement. It also must be administered by pills that spread the drug throughout the body. A better way to inhibit the type 1 5-AR that damages hair growth may be with increased copper ions in the skin. Sugimoto et al found that copper (II) ions could give up to a 90 percent inhibition of type 1 5-AR. At 1.2 micrograms copper ion per milliliter, there was a 50 percent reduction in the activity of type 1 5-AR, but copper (II) ions were 10-fold less active on inhibiting the type 2 prostate form. Thus, copper ions are more specific inhibitors of 5-AR than Propecia. Human transdermal studies have found that concentrations of up to 0.50 micrograms per milliliter centimeter of copper ion can be introduced into the skin with SRCPs without irritation. For comparison, the blood plasma copper level is approximately 1 microgram per milliliter.[4]

Improving microcirculation to hair follicles. Hair follicles have very high rates of metabolic activity. However, morphological studies of aged follicles often find an inadequate capillary circulation, and some researchers have suggested that the resultant lack of nutrient flow may be a causative factor in the thinning of hair shafts with age. SRCPs have angiogenic activity that may correct this problem. See Chapter 16.

Protective anti-inflammatory actions. The final event in the sequence of degenerative changes that produces involuted non-functional hair follicles are tissue-damaging auto-immune inflammatory and free-radical reactions around the follicle. SRCPs may reduce such effects, since they block the inflammatory actions of both Interleukin 1 and Transforming Growth Factor beta 1. Also during tissue injury, the release of ferrous iron from ferritin increases the formation of tissue-damaging free radicals, but SRCPs block the release of iron from ferritin. Finally, copper zinc superoxide dismutase is normally only about 50 percent activated due to a lack of copper in the protein. SRCPs can supply additional copper to zinc superoxide dismutase and increase its antioxidant effectiveness. Autoimmune damage causing hair loss exists in conditions such as alopecia areata, diabetes, vitiligo, certain types of thyroid disease, and pernicious anemia. The treatment for these conditions is usually a short course of any cortisone-type drug, which often restores hair growth. But cortisone injections into the bald spots bring the hair back only temporarily. The problem is that costicosteroids inhibit skin repair and often produce thinner, less functional skin that is less able to support hair follicle functions. In studies on nickel allergic patients, Zhai et al wrote that SRCPs were effective in reducing redness and inflammation after allergic reactions while also stimulating skin repair. See Chapter 16.

Enhancing the skin's subcutaneous fat layer and thickening of the scalp. During human aging, there is a thinning of the scalp. This is partly due to the diminishment of the scalp's subcutaneous fat layer surrounding the hair follicles that occurs with age. Pathologists have noted that large subcutaneous fat cells are associated with large, healthy hair follicles and have postulated that the fat cells provide nutritional support to the follicles. Conditions that cause hair loss, such as cancer chemotherapy, are associated with a sharp decrease in the volume of subcutaneous fat cells. SRCPs increase both the hair follicles' size and the amount of subcutaneous fat. SRCPs also help increase skin thickness by boosting the dermal levels of collagen, elastin, and the water-holding proteoglycans and glycosaminoglycans. See Chapter 16.

Repairing damaged scalp. Hair loss, especially in women, may often be caused by scalp damage from relaxers, permanents, coloring chemicals, and excessive heat from blow dryers and hot oil treatments. SRCPs can be used after various hair procedures to speed the repair of scalp damage.

Reducing graying of hair. Hair becomes gray with age, but the speed at which this happens may depend on the adequacy of available copper in the scalp. Melanin and other hair pigments are produced from the amino acid tyrosine by the action of tyrosinase, a copper-containing enzyme. Additional scalp copper might slow the graying process. Skin Biology clients often report the re-pigmentation of gray hair after using SRCP products.

Using Folligen to Improve Hair Health

Earlier inventions of mine, based on my research in the 1980's, produced products such as Tricomin™, which was demonstrated to increase hair growth in humans, and GraftCyte™, which was proven to increase hair transplant success in humans. For more see Chapter 16. My latest inventions for the hair are Folligen products. Folligen had its beginning as an SRCP skin repair cream that was being tested in the Dermatology Department at the University of California at San Francisco. A 41-year-old woman with severe hair loss tried the skin repair cream on her head because nothing else had worked to restore her lost hair. Over the next two-

> *"And Delilah made Samson sleep upon her knees; and she called for a man, and she caused him to shave off seven locks from Samson's head; and she began to afflict him, and Samson's strength went from him."*
> — *"Capture of Samson", Judges 16*

and-a-half months, she regained all of her lost hair. Word spread, and other people began using the skin repair cream to counter hair loss. In time, Folligen emerged as a distinct product. Folligen's biological effect on hair is similar to my earlier inventions on hair but appears to be more effective in my basic tests on hair function.

Folligen is sold in three versions: Folligen Cream, which works well on hairlines; Folligen Lotion, a more liquid solution for use in areas of denser hair; and Folligen Solution Therapy Spray, which is a fine mist sprayed on the scalp. (There is also a Folligen shampoo and conditioner, which are described at the end of this chapter.)

Folligen products are often used to calm scalp tissue that has been irritated by other hair growth stimulators, such as minoxidil and retinoic acid (Retin-A). When using Folligen for scalp calming, start with a light application. On a very irritated scalp, even Folligen can cause a brief stinging, but as your scalp repairs itself, it will become more protective and less sensitive to irritation by minoxidil, retinoic acid, and other products.

Hair Regrowth Recommendations

Following are recommendations, based on reports from our clients, that may help restore lost or thinning hair. Hair loss in women is normally due to stress or hormonal shifts, such as menopausal changes or stopping the use of birth control pills, and is easier to reverse than hair loss in men.

1. Apply an SRCP product such as Folligen Lotion, Folligen Cream or Folligen Solution Therapy Spray. The recommended use is four to five times a week as a light coating applied before bedtime. Clients usually report that Folligen markedly reduces hair loss in about three weeks, improves scalp health, reduces irritation, and results in a thicker head of hair in about four months.

2. Apply Emu Oil-S for Hair. The combination of Folligen's SRCPs and emu oil often produces drastic reductions in hair loss and increases hair growth. Recently, Dr. Michael Holick of Boston University Medical Center reported a clinical study that found emu oil accelerated skin regeneration and also stimulated hair growth. He wrote, "The hair follicles were more robust, the skin thickness was remarkably increased…Also, we discovered in the same test that over 80 percent of hair follicles that had been 'asleep' were awakened and began growing hair."

3. For added stimulation, apply minoxidil (2 to 5 percent). Start by using 2 percent minoxidil. This can be progressively increased to 5 percent minoxidil. Sometimes minoxidil produces scalp irritation. If this happens, stop using the product and only use Folligen until your scalp health is restored. Then, resume the use of 2 percent minoxidil, and eventually 5 percent minoxidil if your scalp remains healthy.

Hideo Uno, who wrote the textbook on Rogaine®, found that both SRCPs and minoxidil work to improve hair health. While minoxidil primarily stimulates new vellus hair growth, SRCPs are more effective in thickening the hair shafts.

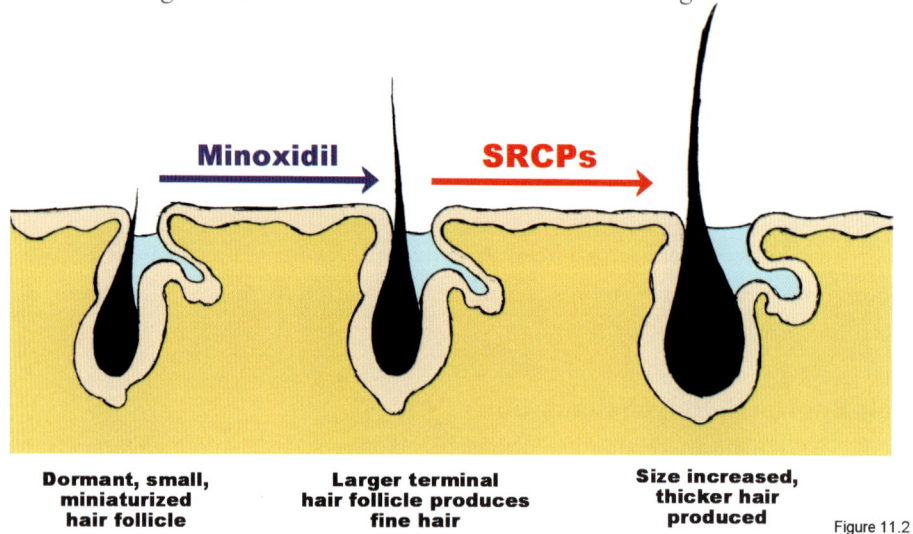

Dormant, small, miniaturized hair follicle → **Minoxidil** → **Larger terminal hair follicle produces fine hair** → **SRCPs** → **Size increased, thicker hair produced**

Figure 11.2

4. Added stimulation can also be found by applying retinoic acid (0.01 to 0.05 percent). Retinoic acid helps produce thicker hair shafts when combined with minoxidil, but this combination may cause scalp irritation. When used lightly, Folligen can greatly reduce the irritation.

5. Women whose hair thins or falls out as the result of a drop in estrogen, such as that which occurs with menopause, can benefit from estrogen supplementation. This raises the estrogen level and helps restore the emotional and physical condition of the woman to the pre-menopausal state. While hormone replacement therapy has been a controversial treatment for menopause, newer methods are finding overall reductions both in the risk of some cancers and in the risk of heart disease. The best-known DHT blocker is Propecia; however, its maker (Merck) does not recommend Propecia for women. In addition, a one-year study of hair growth in 136 post-menopausal women found no significant effect of Propecia on hair growth.

6. For those who prefer an all-natural approach, there are several non-drug DHT blockers. These include saw palmetto oil, pygeum and nettle root extract, the soybean isoflavones genistein and daidzein, ginkgo biloba, and gamma linoleic acid.

Saw palmetto oil has been used for more than 400 years as an herbal treatment for enuresis, nocturia, atrophy of the testes, impotence, inflammation of the prostate, and as a mild aphrodisiac for men. Women used the berries to treat infertility, painful periods, and problems with lactation. Extracts of two plants, pygeum bark (Pygeum africanum) and nettle root (Urtica dioica) are widely used for the treatment of prostate hyperplasia.

Isoflavonoids, such as genistein and daidzein, are weak estrogens and may lessen the risk of osteoporosis and heart disease. Several studies have found a protective effect of isoflavones against the development of cancer. The Chinese report that daidzien exhibits hair-growth and hair-color-promoting activity.

Ginkgo biloba is a popular herb used worldwide to improve cerebral blood flow and general blood circulation.

Getting Rid of Any Green

Blond hair may pick up a green tint when exposed to Folligen. This is similar to the greenish tint that may occur after spending time in a swimming pool. Try to keep the products on the scalp. If a green tint occurs, a solution of one part lemon juice and four parts water will remove the green color. A tin-peptide product (such as Folligen for Blondes) has no color problems and often works to reduce hair loss.

Folligen Shampoo and Conditioner

Folligen Therapy Shampoo and Folligen Therapy Conditioner are relatively low pH products and are designed to clean the hair with the minimum amount of damage, then tighten up and re-seal the hair shafts. SRCPs are added to enhance the vitality of the hair follicles and scalp.

Hair has a high sulfur content from the amino acid cysteine and can easily form cross-links to other cystines in the hair molecule. These bonds are responsible for the hair's toughness and abrasion resistance. The cross-links hold the hair fibers together. As long as this organization is not disrupted, the fiber is strong and appears "healthy".

Shampoos of more (higher) alkaline pH may work better to clean the hair and scalp, but they also strip away too many natural scalp oils and extract the "glues" that help hold the hair shafts together. Folligen Therapy Shampoo doesn't contain "flash-foamers", or foaming chemicals that add lather (which does nothing for the hair and damages the hair shafts and scalp).

Folligen Therapy Conditioner is formulated to re-acidify the hair after shampooing. Restoring this natural acid environment to the hair and scalp helps keep the hair proteins hard and prevents the growth of foreign bacteria. The conditioner contains the highest-quality amino acids and pantothenic acid (vitamin B-5) to re-seal the hair cuticle after shampooing. It is designed to help de-tangle the hair and add a lustrous shine. SRCPs are added to help enhance the health and vitality of the hair, scalp, and hair follicles.

Because Folligen Therapy Shampoo and Folligen Therapy Conditioner are concentrated, you may want to mix the products with a small amount of water to make them easier to use.

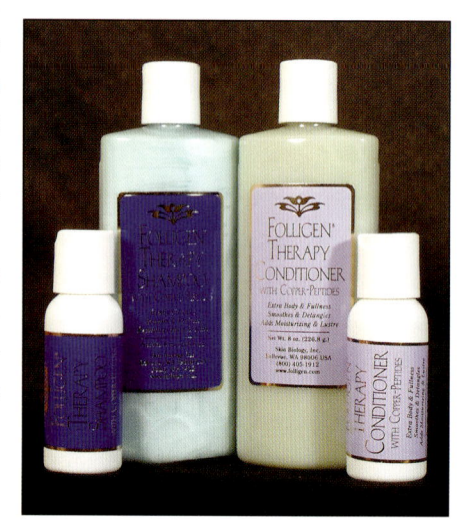

Testimonials

"Update on my husband. He was and still is, using minoxodil 5%, and introduced diluted CP Serum about three months ago, switching to Folligen and also adding nizoral twice a week in the last month. He has new growth along the hairline, and in some spots the hair is black at the roots and grey at the tip. My kids were amazed with that…He is very impressed."-K

"I have been using Folligen Spray (applied with a dropper), Emu Oil for hair and Folligen Shampoo for the last 3 and 1/2 months. I was applying the Folligen Spray every day until SkinBio reported better results with every other day application. Since then I am following their recommendation…The reason I started using CPs on my hair was to get a healthier scalp, not for baldness. But the hair on the top of my head was less thick than the rest of it. So, after more than 3 months I am noticing a lot of new growth. It is quite visible since I had a tuft of white hair and the new growth is dark and shorter…It is a lot of fun to see all those new hairs, and dark too! I also notice my hair grows faster; I need to have a hair cut more often."-M

"I have NEW hair!! LOL, I was looking in the mirror yesterday and noticed I had new hairs growing around my hairline. They are about one inch long, yippee…I've been using Folligen Cream sporadically and then more consistently for the last 3 weeks or so. About three weeks ago I started using some minoxidil sort of regularly about the same time I started using the Folligen more regularly. I'm excited! Just last week I ordered the Folligen Shampoo and Conditioner and now I'm really motivated to be good about using everything on a regular consistent basis and see what happens."-S

Chapter 12

Biology, Chemistry, And Hair Care

Throughout history, hair has been an important part of romantic and sexual attraction. Mermaids and sirens of the sea and the maiden Lorelei of the river Rhine are said to have brought men to disaster who became transfixed by the beauty of their long tresses. Australian aborigines saved their wives' hair clippings as a prized possession. Even today, some orthodox Jewish women only allow their husbands to see their hair.

Although different cultures desire different qualities in hair, most people are attracted to hair that is relatively dense, thick stranded, strongly pigmented and (for a woman) somewhat long. As with the skin, the "ideal" hair closely approximates the physical characteristics of the hair of a young child. Sadly, as we age, our hair moves away from that ideal by becoming damaged, thinning and losing pigment. However, proper hair care can reduce, and in some cases even reverse, the effects of the passing years.

What Is Hair?

Hair is a specialized form of skin, as are nails, scales, feathers, horns, and claws. Although the hair on the head generally gets the most attention, hair grows over a large percentage of the human body, serving protective, sensory, and sexual attractiveness functions.

A single hair has a thickness of 0.02 to 0.04 millimeters, so 20 to 50 hair fibers next to one other span about one millimeter. Humans have about five million hairs on our bodies, with about 450,000 of them found above the neck. Most people have about 150,000 hairs on their head and normally shed 25 to 100 hairs a day while growing an equivalent number of new hairs. Another 30,000 hairs reside in men's mustaches and beards. Blondes usually have more scalp hair than those with dark or red hair.

> "If a woman has long hair, it is a glory unto her."
> — St. Paul, I Corinthians

Mature hairs are filaments composed primarily of proteins (88 percent) of a hard, tough, fibrous type known as keratin. Proteins are built up from individual amino acids to form long chains where each amino acid is a link in the chain. The keratin found in human hair is also a major protein in fingernails. Hair has a very hard outer coating, the Cuticle, consisting of overlapping scale-like bits of hard keratin. The inside or cortex is a core of softer protein filaments.

Hair proteins have a high sulfur content from the amino acid cysteine, which forms cross-links in the hair proteins that are responsible for the hair's toughness and abrasion resistance. You would never guess when looking at all the hairs that collect in your brush, but human hair is as strong as a wire of iron. But it rips after being damaged or stretched 70 percent beyond its original length.

The Hair's Many Hues

The shades of human hair are too numerous to count and range from black to brown and red to blonde. Hair color is partly influenced by how light bounces off the hair proteins, but is primarily determined by the type and amount of pigment contained within the hair shaft center. Eumelanin is the pigment found in black and brown hair and to a lesser degree in blonde hair. Pheomelanin produces red hair, while a mix of eumelanin and pheomelanin produces the blonde-red combination known as strawberry blonde. The greater the amount of pigment in the hair, the darker the hair color. As the amount of pigment is reduced, the hair color turns from black to brown and then reddish or blond. If pigment is significantly diminished, the hair appears gray, and if it is absent, the hair becomes white.

As we age, our hair color generally changes. Many "towheaded" children who have blonde-whitish hair as youngsters turn into brunette adults and eventually gray or white-haired elders.

Under some circumstances, the hair can lose its color prematurely. One of these is severe stress. For example, in the trench warfare of World War I, there were cases of young men whose hair turned gray within two months after prolonged episodes of severe fighting and artillery bombardments. Another cause of prematurely gray or white hair is malnutrition; a lack of sufficient dietary copper can cause the hair to lose its color. Excessive dietary zinc may drive out the copper needed to synthesize hair pigments and turn hair gray.

Hair Length and Growth

Hair grows faster in the spring and summer, a fact that is often manipulated to "prove" that certain hair-growth remedies are effective. In actuality, the rate at which the hair grows is dependent on the individual and his or her age, diet, and so on. The length of time your hair follicles stay in the anagen phase is responsible for determining the maximum length your hair will grow. On average, waist-length hair takes about five years to grow out from a short haircut, periodic trims included. Following is a list of average lengths and growth rates of the hair on the head and body.

Hairs:	Average length (cm)	Growth rate per day (mm)
On the head	70	0.35
Eyebrows	1.0	0.15
Mustaches (beards or whiskers)	28	0.4
Armpit hairs	5	0.3
Pubic hairs	4	0.2

Factors that Damage Hair

Hair fibers can be damaged by many different factors, including environmental elements (such as prolonged exposure to sunlight or wind) and chemical and mechanical injuries (such as tight hairstyles, hot rollers, hot oil treatments, and harsh use of hair dryers). The chemicals used to alter hair, including bleaches, dyes, relaxers, and perming agents, all cause varying degrees of damage. Some cosmetic products partially repair damaged hair, but a good quality of hair will return only after the production of new hair.

The Damaging Things We Do
TO OUR HAIR

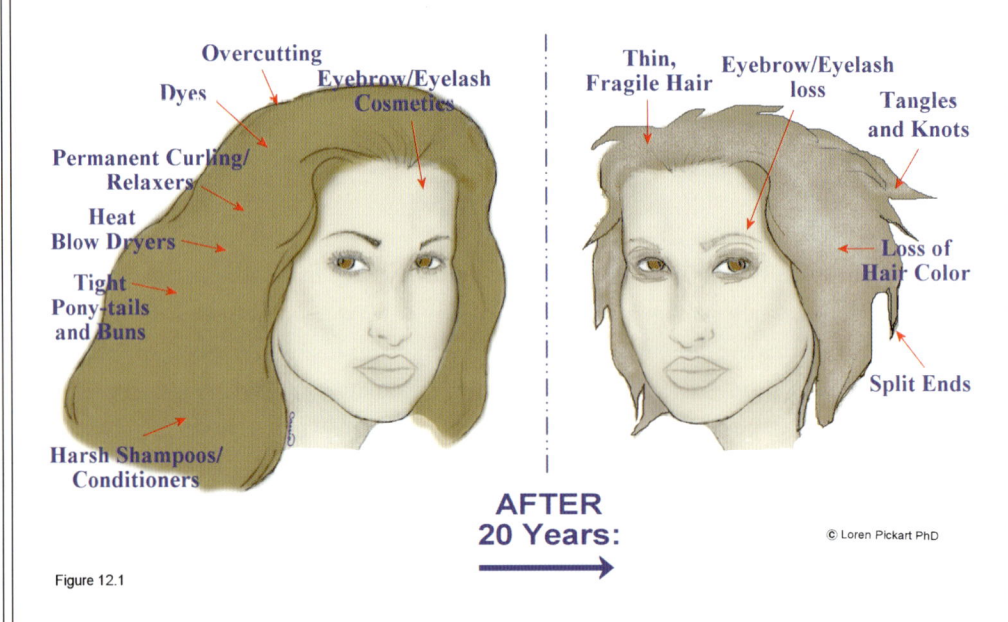

Before (left): Dyes, Overcutting, Eyebrow/Eyelash Cosmetics, Permanent Curling/Relaxers, Heat Blow Dryers, Tight Pony-tails and Buns, Harsh Shampoos/Conditioners

AFTER 20 Years: Thin, Fragile Hair, Eyebrow/Eyelash loss, Tangles and Knots, Loss of Hair Color, Split Ends

© Loren Pickart PhD

Figure 12.1

Choosing the Right Shampoo

Excessive shampooing is the main cause of damage to the hair shafts. It is important to choose your shampoo carefully. The best shampoos are around pH 6.0, at the high end of the slightly acid pH of the scalp (4.5 to 6.0). Maintaining the natural acid environment of the hair and scalp keeps the hair proteins hard and prevents the growth of foreign bacteria. Preserving the natural hair and skin oils helps protect scalp health.

Shampoos with a higher pH have a negative effect on the hair for several reasons. While more alkaline shampoos work better to clean the hair and scalp, they also strip away many of the hair's natural oils and the "glues" that help hold the hair shafts together. A high pH shampoo may make your hair look great for a few weeks, but eventually it will cause your hair to become dry and brittle and lead to increased breakage.

Don't be fooled by baby shampoos, which are formulated for gentleness if they get in the eyes. Many baby shampoos have a high pH. Also be careful of "clarifying shampoos". Formulated to remove materials that build up on the hair, such as mousse and hair spray, they can also remove color and perms. Some hair experts recommend using a combination of plain baking soda and your normal shampoo to remove build-up. Other ingredients to avoid include flash foamers, chemicals that enhance the foaming effect of shampoo, and added fragrances, neither of which have a positive effect.

Choosing the right shampoo is especially important for those with oily hair. This type of hair is more difficult to manage than normal or dry hair and is often tough to comb. Oily hair is covered with sebum from the sebaceous glands of the hair follicle. Frequent washing with a stronger, more-soapy shampoo helps remove oil but can damage the hair. Some Skin Biology clients with oily hair use retinoic acid to reduce oil production. Retinoic acid should be used sparingly, as overuse can result in scalp irritation.

Don't choose a shampoo based on an expensive price tag. A shampoo's price is generally related to the cost of its advertising. If the label on a shampoo bottle tells you to wash your hair twice, ignore it; the manufacturer is simply encouraging you to use more of the product. Always use a minimum amount of shampoo. Some shampoo manufacturers recommend that you comb through wet hair to distribute the shampoo evenly. But wet hair is more easily broken, and you will only end up with damaged hair.

When you are done washing your hair, the shampoo should be completely rinsed out to help bring the pH back down to its natural level. If your hair is very dry, only shampoo every three days. Our ancestors went months between hair washings, one of the reasons their hair was so healthy.

Choosing the Right Conditioner

The outer layer of hair called the cuticle is somewhat like fish scales made of hard keratin. The cuticle is held together by disulfide bonds plus small amino acids. In healthy hair, the outer layer of scales lies flat; the hair looks shiny and combs and brushes glide smoothly through it. Hair with damaged cuticle appears dry, drab, split, brittle, or frizzy.

Quality conditioners add amino acids, peptides, and pantothenic acid (vitamin B-5) into the cuticle to help glue the scales tightly to the hair shaft. If the cuticle stays open, it can start a tear in the hair shaft that leads to breakage of the shaft.

Quality conditioners have a low pH of about 4.0 to 4.7. The hair proteins remain hard and strong at a low pH. Some conditioners contain a small amount of fat to give the hair a better shine. The best products are sold in successful hair salons. These salons need happy, repeat customers and usually do not advertise their products. The longer you leave the conditioner on your hair, the better it works. Some manufacturers recommend leaving conditioner on the hair for only a few seconds, but longer is generally better (one to two minutes).

Many of the conditioners on the market today contain botanicals, such as extracts of juniper berries and buckhorn leaves. These ingredients should be avoided. Herbal extracts interfere with the glue process and reduce the protective effects of the conditioner. Also beware of combs with unpolished teeth, sharp hair clamps, and tight elastic bands, all of which can disrupt the hair scales.

Shampoos, Conditioners, and SRCPs
(Skin Remodeling Copper-Peptides)

Why your hair needs a separate Shampoo & Conditioner...

INSIDE:
Cortex is the soft center of hair shaft.

Cuticle is the outer hard, overlapping scales of protein.

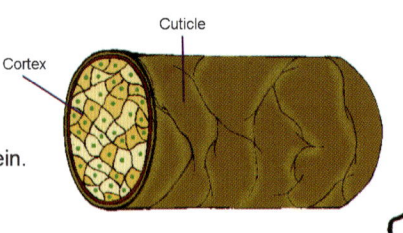

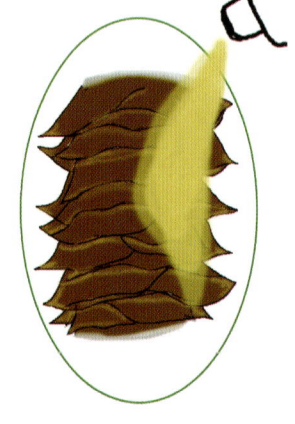

1. Damaged hair has open cuticle that causes ripping, tearing, and breakage. Use a mild shampoo and rinse well.

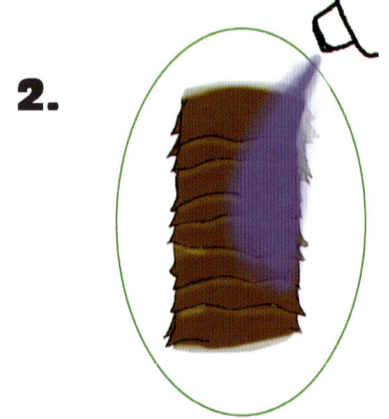

2. Follow with acid conditioner to harden and flatten cuticle and apply protective nutrients.

3. Over a period of time, hair shaft lies flat providing sealed hair shaft with protective proteins that prevent growth of bacteria, split ends, help detangle, and add a lustrous shine to the hair.

SRCPs also help calm the scalp.

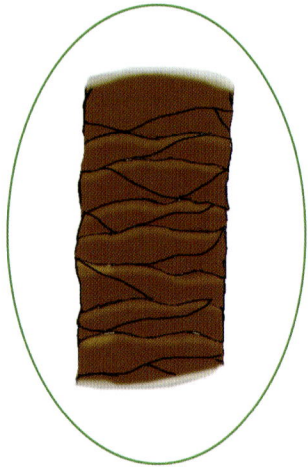

Figure 12-2
© Loren Pickart PhD

Never use a combination or 2-in-1 shampoo/conditioner

The Benefits of Regular Brushing

Brushing your hair every day keeps your scalp healthy and improves the blood circulation that feeds the hair follicles. Regular brushing also helps distribute the protective and lubricating fats along the length of the hair shafts.

There is a formula to proper brushing. A natural-bristle brush works best because it is similar to the hair structure and less likely to produce tangles in long hair. The brush should have a wooden base to reduce static electricity. If combing, start with a wide-tooth tortoiseshell comb. Never use a metal or rubber comb. Stand with your feet a little apart and bend from the waist until your hair falls in a curtain in front of your face.

Brush the hair gently, starting from the roots at the nape of the neck and moving toward the end of the hair. Follow each brush stroke with a stroke from the open palm of your other hand to help counteract the buildup of static electricity. Continue for 50 strokes. Repeat once a day.

Tips for Long, Healthy Hair

The famous hair stylist George Michael mentioned in the last chapter (now retired and living in Florida) is known for his methods of helping women grow out their hair to very long lengths. Dr. Michael believes that longer hair is healthier hair, or as he puts it, "The longer the hair, the stronger the root." Many women are taught that by age 30, their hair should be no longer than shoulder length. Dr. Michael feels the opposite is true. He believes long hair is majestic on a mature woman--that it downplays wrinkles and makes her look younger.

When counseling women on how to grow their hair long, Dr. Michael taught them that it is important to have hair that is all one length, without bangs or layers. According to his findings, the body tries to equalize uneven hair by excessively shedding strands.

Longer Hair Reduces Shedding - Studies by Dr. George Michael	
Hair Length - inches	Number Hairs Lost Per Day
4	87
12	26
Waist Length	16
Floor Length	2

When working with long-haired clients, Dr. Michael had many methods of protecting the hair. He used hair dryers set only about 10 degrees F higher than body temperature (most blow dryers reach temperatures of up to 260 degrees and damage hair follicles). When curling the hair, he used large rollers of soft mesh or plastic rather than rollers that grab the hair, which can tear the hair. Special care was taken to protect the ends of the hair when rolling or setting. Shampoos were kept to a minimum. Vitamin and mineral supplements were recommended. Dr. Michael also recommended covering the hair at all times when exposed to direct sunlight. (See www.longhairlovers.com).

Hair Experts' Suggestions for Long, Healthy Hair
1. Hair is best cut when dry.

2. Detangle dry hair before washing. Detangle the ends first and work your way up. Do not try to remove tangles from top to bottom since this may pull out hair. Before entering the shower, give your hair a few strokes with a comb or brush. This aligns the strands and helps prevent tangles.

3. When washing your hair, use water at room temperature. The lower the temperature of the water, the better it is for your hair. Warm water opens the hair scales, making the hair shaft more vulnerable to damage.

4. When preparing to wash your hair, bring the hair in front of your face before wetting it and leave it there. Let your hair hang down in front during shampooing. Try not to move your hair while you wash it. This keeps the hair strands in position so they won't move upwards and wrap themselves around other strands, resulting in tangles.

5. Don't try to "wash" your hair. The purpose of shampoo is to remove dirt from the top layers. Just let the shampoo penetrate the lower layers briefly as it flows over your hair.

6. Make sure to wash out all of the shampoo. When you think all of the shampoo is gone, allow another half-minute of constant water flow to ensure that the residue is gone. For a final rinse, use cool or cold water.

7. Use an acidifying conditioner with peptides to re-glue the protein scales of the cuticle. Put extra conditioner on your hair ends to prevent split ends. Give the conditioner at least a minute to glue into the hair. For a final rinse, use cool or cold water.

8. Air-dry your hair whenever possible.

9. When you must blow-dry your hair, first wrap it in a special, highly absorbent towel to remove water. Blow-dry the hair for a few minutes, and then let it air dry. A cool setting on the hair dryer helps "set" the hair.

10. Never use a heavy-duty reconstructor on your hair. It does more harm than good.

11. Excessive sunlight and use of tanning beds harms the hair.

12. Use a non-alcohol hair spray, which is less drying.

13. Use wide-toothed combs and picks.

14. Only use coated or snag-free elastics and hair fasteners.

15. Think of your hair as a silk garment and treat it accordingly. Both silk and hair are protein fibers. You wouldn't wash a silk garment with a cheap detergent in a washing machine at a high temperature with a high agitation cycle and then dry it in a dryer at a high temperature.

16. Many hairdressers only "cut" hair. For long hair, tell them to keep trimming to an absolute minimum. Avoid hyper-critical hairdressers.

17. If someone criticizes your hair, ignore them. Hair arouses many emotions and jealousies, so arrange your hair in a fashion that pleases yourself.

Changing the Look of Your Hair

Your hair's appearance can be altered by changing its shape through permanent waving or straightening. However, both of these procedures cause damage to the scalp and hair. This damage might include breakage, thinning, lack of hair growth, scalp irritation, scalp damage, and hair loss. If the damage becomes excessive, serious hair loss may occur.

The following is information about both procedures. Before undergoing any hair treatment, especially one that introduces powerful chemicals to your hair, you owe it to yourself to be well informed.

Permanents

Permanents break the disulfide bonds in the proteins that hold hair together to allow the hair to be wrapped around a roller and formed into a new texture. Then the disulfide bonds are chemically reset and the new, curly texture is locked into place. But when the perming solution is left on too long, is too strong, or is applied to hair that has already been damaged by dye, bleach, or an earlier perm, the hair and hair follicles can be severely damaged. If this happens to you, rub Folligen Lotion into your scalp for three to four nights following the procedure to restore scalp health.

Hair Straightening

Hair straightening is increasingly popular. During the procedure, disulfide bonds that keep hair curly are broken by an alkaline-reducing agent. Hair relaxers are typically creams or cream lotions containing about 2 to 4 percent of strong bases such as sodium hydroxide, potassium hydroxide, and lithium hydroxide or 5 percent calcium hydroxide plus a solution of up to about 30 percent guanidine carbonate. The pH is around 12. Some relaxers contain about 4 percent ammonium thioglycolate as the active ingredient.

Before the straightening procedure, a petroleum-base cream is applied to the hair to help protect the scalp. Then the relaxer chemical is applied and the hair is combed straight. After a period of time, the chemical is removed with warm water and a neutralizing formula. Finally, a conditioner is applied to the hair to restore some of the natural oils and proteins removed by the chemical.

As with perms, the harsh chemicals used in hair straightening can cause severe damage to the hair. The procedure should be followed with applications of Folligen Lotion to restore scalp health.

Hair straightening should only be done by a hair-care professional with a record of success in chemical straightening. It is strongly recommended that you obtain professional conditioning treatments before and after the process.

Alternatively, intense heat can also reset hair bonds, allowing curly hair to be straightened with a flat iron, or even by ironing with a regular electric iron and an ironing board or flat surface covered with a smooth towel. But extreme heat is also very damaging to the hair.

Chemical Hair Relaxers

His name was Garrett Augustus Morgan, and he was born the seventh of 11 children of former slaves. He is best known for his invention of the automatic traffic signal and gas mask. Around 1910, while attempting to invent a new lubricating liquid for the sewing machine, Morgan wiped his hands on a wool cloth and found that the woolly texture of the cloth became "smoothed out." He experimented on his curly haired Airedale dog, and the effect was successfully duplicated. Morgan called his discovery a "hair-refining cream" and patented the first chemical hair relaxer.

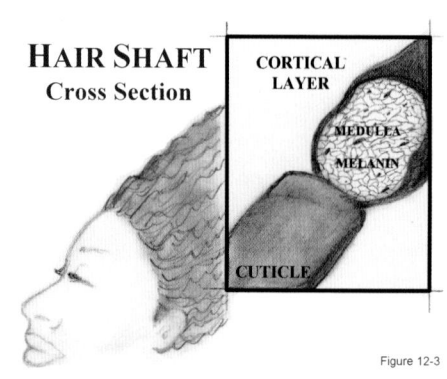

Figure 12-3

Today Morgan's discovery, lye (sodium hydroxide), is still a common ingredient in chemical relaxers because it provides the strongest and most dramatic effect. But this same ingredient is also found in strong drain cleaners.

Guanidine hydroxide is another chemical commonly found in hair relaxers. Often referred to as the "no-lye" relaxer, the name doesn't mean that there isn't a strong chemical at work. Although this type of relaxer can be less damaging than its counterpart, the hair and scalp should still be in top condition before attempting the procedure.

How Chemical Relaxers Work

How can chemicals "relax" or straighten hair? Both lye and no-lye relaxers are very strong chemicals that work in the same manner by changing the basic structure of the hair shaft. The chemical penetrates the cortex or cortical layer and loosens the natural curl pattern. However, this inner layer of the hair shaft not only gives curly hair its shape, it also provides strength and elasticity. Once the straightening process is performed, it is irreversible. The result is straighter hair, but hair that is much weaker and more susceptible to breaking.

"Over-processing," the excessive use of relaxers on the hair or applying the chemical to already processed or relaxed hair, is the most typical misuse of hair-relaxing chemicals. Once the initial relaxer is applied to "virgin hair" (or a "virgin relaxer" is performed), touch-ups should only be applied to new growth no more than every six to eight weeks.

Hair Removal Techniques for Women and Men

Surveys indicate that 80 percent of women and more than 50 percent of men have unwanted hair in various body areas. Much of this unwanted hair is genetic, but sometimes it is the result of other causes, such as testosterone treatment. Those looking to get rid of unwanted hair have several options, described as follows.

– Tweezing, Shaving, Mechanical Epilators, Chemical Depilatories
– Less Hair Eventually: Waxing (tends to reduce hair growth with time)
– Permanent: Electrolysis (Hair Electrology), Laser Hair Removal

Shaving 101

The most popular method of hair removal is shaving. Since shaving is temporary and must be repeated often, proper shaving is important. Before shaving, wash the skin to exfoliate the skin and lift the hair away from the follicle; this softens the hair and prepares it for the shave. When shaving, shave in the same direction each time (down rather than up); this helps train the hair to grow out straight, making for an easier shave.

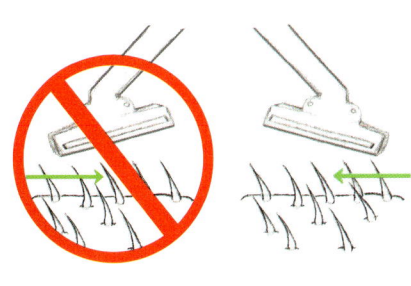

Figure 12-4

You may notice that, not long after you shave, small bumps appear. These may become further irritated, resulting in redness, itchiness, discoloration, or infection. The bumps are pseudofolliculitis barbae, commonly referred to as "ingrown hairs" or "razor bumps." Many people have found a decrease in ingrown hairs when using an electric razor, although the shave may not be as close as that of a blade. Exfoliating and cleansing the face is your best defense against ingrown hairs and razor bumps. Recommended exfoliating agents include Skin Biology's Exfol Serum or Exfol Cream. Gentle cleansing and keeping the skin smooth and supple works well to keep the hair follicles moisturized and growing in the right direction.

The Importance of Skin Healing After Hair Removal

All hair-removal methods (tweezing, shaving, waxing, electrolysis, lasers, pharmaceutical creams, and so on) cause skin damage that allows for the penetration of viruses and bacteria into the skin. For example, warts seem to start from injured or broken skin. In adults, warts tend to grow where hair-removal procedures have damaged the skin, such as the beard area of men and the legs of women. To restore the skin after shaving, many Skin Biology clients apply BioHeal. The cream closes the skin's surface to viruses and bacteria and helps heal the skin.

Longer Eyelashes, Thicker Eyebrows

The loss of eyebrows and eyelashes is often due to long-term use of cosmetics. However, some have reported a reversal of this effect through the light use of an SRCP product. We recommend trying a light application of Folligen Cream followed by Emu Oil-S.

This often helps restore the lost hairs in about two months. For eyebrows: each day apply Folligen Cream then Emu Oil-S for Hair. For eyelashes: Each day apply a light coating of Folligen Cream and Emu Oil-S for Hair to the skin below or above the eyelashes, near the "eyelash bed" (where the eyelashes would protrude from).

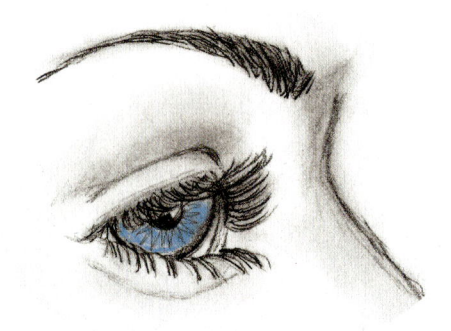

Figure 12.5

Testimonials:

"I put some Folligen on my eyelashes, because I seem to lose a few every week, and after 2 weeks, they are much longer and thicker and curling upwards... I started applying Folligen, because I used to lose a lash or two each week, not that it was noticeable, but just found them on my cheek.

Since I started applying Folligen, none have fallen out... I am using a tiny amount, by the way, just enough to be able to spread across the lash line. I do both upper and lower... Mine are definitely longer, not just thicker, and in just 3.5 weeks I would say at least 10-20% longer." - D

"I have been using cp for 4 months now and I too have noticed my eyebrow hair thickening. In fact they are wrapping around thicker all the time. So not only is my skin younger looking but my eyebrows are younger looking also." - GH

"I've been using CP Night Eyes, CP Serum, Exfol, and P&R for about one month... I did notice about two weeks ago when I put on Mascara that WOW my lashes were looking very good! The mascara was the same as always so I can only assume that the lashes are changing. I have noticed more length and possibly thickening. In any case, I certainly like this added benefit." - BRG

"Must say my eyebrows & lashes are looking so much thicker I am very happy about that." - MY

"My light eyebrows are definitely getting darker! I am elated!" - JN

"After many years of using eye makeup and eye makeup remover I've noticed that my lashes are no longer as thick as they once were. I have been using the follicle creme and emu oil [Folligen Cream and Emu Oil-S for Hair] on my lashes... it seems that my eyelashes are thicker. I believe that I am no longer losing lashes like I use to.

Also, my husband has a little bald spot the size of a nickle. The loss of hair was due to stress and has never grown back. I am applying the creme along with the emu oil on it nightly. So far it appears that thin blond hairs are starting to grow... We're both really impressed with your products." - NL

> *"I will be arriving in Paris tomorrow evening. Don't Wash!"*
> — Napoleon (Message to Josephine)

Chapter 13

The Formula of Love

Have you ever noticed how when a teenager enters the room, all eyes are drawn to him or her? This is a testament to the power of pheromones, chemical substances produced by humans, animals, and plants that serves as a stimulus to others. Research shows that human pheromones may be responsible for a host of behaviors, ranging from mothers kissing their children to men being attracted to large-breasted women.

The human pheromone level peaks at around age 18, and then slowly declines throughout our lives. When we enter a room at age 40, our pheromone signal no longer excites others as it did when we were 18. People tend to assume that the physical beauty of young people is the sole source of their attractiveness without considering that smells also activate emotions. Perhaps the declining interest of others as we age is not only due to the physical changes in our bodies, but also to the decline in our pheromones. As a result, the most effective way for aging individuals to attract attention may be to enhance their natural pheromone signal with supplemental pheromones, just as we take supplements of antioxidants to keep healthy and ward off disease.[1]

The Two Types of Pheromones

While the effects of pheromones on humans are less obvious than in other mammals, they still strongly affect our behavior. As pheromones move among us, they activate pre-coded genetic programs.

Pheromones fall into two categories. The first is signal pheromones, airborne particles that pass through the air after being evaporated by the heat of the body. When you wear clothes, your body heats the air, causing it to rise toward the highest opening. As the heated air rises, it picks up the pheromones secreted from your skin. As the air emerges around your face, it causes people to look at and notice you. It takes about one second for smells from your face to reach someone 50 feet away in still air. In addition to making others aware of our presence, signal pheromones also cause immediate changes in behavior by activating certain areas of the brain.

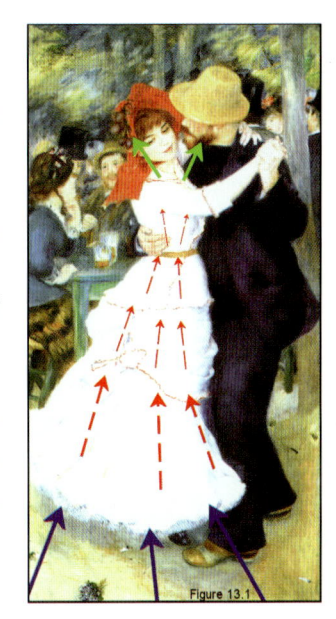

Figure 13.1

The second type of pheromone is priming pheromones, heavy proteins that are passed by kissing or skin-to-skin contact. This may be why kissing occurs in all human cultures; as a way of passing pheromones. When a mother kisses her baby, for instance, it increases mother-baby bonding. Priming pheromones increase the production of many hormones that effect development, metabolism, and mating behavior. Consider how sometimes, fertile women have difficulty becoming pregnant. In married couples, it takes an average of six months of sexual intercourse to produce the first pregnancy. One theory is that the woman's body must slowly adjust to her husband's pheromones before becoming receptive to pregnancy. The desire for being held and cuddled is very strong in women—something a new husband quickly learns can help him have a smooth relationship with his wife.

Why Women Call Men "Pigs"

In goats, sheep, pigs, and some other animals, male competition for females is determined by the strength of the male's pheromones rather than physical strength or beauty. The animals with the strongest pheromones have more confident threat displays without giving signals of fear. This reduces the incidence of actual physical combat for females, especially among deer and moose. The signal of the male with the strongest pheromones causes a psychological castration of the other males that helps remove them from competition.

This type of pheromone dominance may also apply to humans. Many researchers think human pheromone responses are very similar to those of pigs. As hard as this may be on the ego, it's probably true. Consider how truffles, a fungus that grows underground near oak trees in France and Italy, have long been highly valued as a human aphrodisiac. Pigs, too, are passionately attracted to truffles and are used to locate the precious fungi. Another indicator is the way women often call men "pigs." On the other hand, men very rarely use this term when talking about women. One explanation is that since the domestication of wild pigs 7,000 years ago, women have intuitively known that many male human hormones are similar to those of pigs. So if you are a man, your pheromone smell may affect females more strongly than your good looks, money, or wit.

> "The purest union that can exist between a man and a woman is that caused by the sense of smell and is sanctioned by the brain's normal assimilation of the animate molecules emitted by the secretions produced by two bodies in contact and sympathy, and in their subsequent evaporation."
> – Auguste Galopin

The key pheromone in pigs is androstenone, which gives boar urine its characteristic odor and is also responsible for some of the odor in human male urine. Female pigs are extremely aware of the smell of androstenone, as are human females to male smells. Pig breeders spray androstenone from aerosol cans on the backs of female pigs to determine whether the female is ready for breeding; if the sow arches her back, she is sexually receptive.

Smells Affect Our Emotions

During the Middle Ages, a man would wipe his brow after dancing and present the cloth to his lady as a love token. The reason for this behavior may not have been consciously realized, but it meant that the lady would have her man's smell with her. The wives of Welsh miners working the night shift would put their man's nightshirts in their pillows where they could smell them. Even today, women often like to wear unwashed T-shirts previously worn by men. Such is the power of scent.

Current theories postulate that smells affect the brain's emotional control areas by activating nerves in the vomero-nasal organ (VMO) in the nasal septum. To understand the influence of smell on the brain, it helps to understand how the brain works. There are three general areas of the brain. The first and most basic is the brain stem, which controls functions such as breathing and heartbeat. The second area is the limbic system in the central area of the brain, the place where intense emotions arise. Some limbic areas cause feelings of peace, contentment, and attraction, while other areas cause feelings of anger, rage, hostility, loneliness, and so on. The conscious brain is the topmost and outer area of the brain. This is where thinking occurs. However, the conscious mind is not where our emotions are developed. The reason we love someone has more to do with how he or she smells to the limbic system than what we consciously think. The signals from smells are sent directly to the limbic system where emotions arise.

Pheromones affect how we feel about and react to others from the moment we are born. Newborn infants follow the breast odors emanating from their mother's nipple/areola region. These odors exert a pheromone effect that guides the infant to nurse at his mother's nipples. Within minutes of birth, the mother's breast odor causes the baby's head to turn and helps guide the baby to successful suckling of milk. These nipple pheromones may also explain the irrational obsession of men with women's breasts. It may be that this is a natural bonding pheromone that men require for their emotional stability and helps tie them to women.[2]

> "Her breasts, like lilies, 'ere their leaves be shed;
> Her nipples, like young blossomed jessamines;
> Such fragrant flowers do give most odorous smell.
> But her sweet odour did them all excell."
> – Edmund Spencer

Since smells have such a powerful impact on our emotions, it comes as no surprise that a lack of smell limits emotional attachment. Approximately 1.3 percent of the population is born with a total lack of smell, known as anosmia. Persons with anosmia often complain about a lack of libido. While they may marry, emotional distance remains a problem. Likewise, the decline in sex drive with aging coincides with the decline in smell.

Pheromones Act Even if You Can't Smell Them

While many pheromones have distinct smells, both animals and humans may be influenced by a small amount of a pheromone that is not large enough to create a conscious odor. For example, a male dog can respond to pheromones from a female dog at a distance of up to three miles, at a concentration the dog is unlikely to consciously smell.

Humans also respond to pheromone levels that are too low to smell. At Stanford University, Sobel and colleagues found that an airborne fragrant pheromone (oestra-1,3,5(10),16-tetraen-3yl acetate) activated brain centers even when present at concentrations below a threshold of conscious detection.[3]

Bathing and the Decline of Bonding

As cultures advance to higher levels of bathing, interpersonal bonding seems to decline. This suggests that washing removes skin pheromones and weakens interpersonal bonding in families and between couples.

The tie between washing and the decline of bonding is present throughout history, from ancient to modern times. In the Roman Republic, family ties were very strong. However, as this society evolved into the wealthy Roman Empire, with its adequate water supplies and free municipal baths, personal bonds became weaker, divorce became common, and social disorganization increased. With the rise of Christianity, with its dislike of nudity and bathing, family ties began to strengthen.

In the United States, California led the way in personal cleanliness. By the 1940's, many Californians bathed or showered daily, washing away their personal pheromones in the process, while most of the U.S. stuck to weekly bathing. California soon led the nation in divorce rates and family breakdown. Likewise, in Europe,

Scandinavia led the way in personal cleanliness in the 20th century and soon experienced family breakdown and chronic cultural complaints of interpersonal coldness. Immense social programs, prosperous economies, and a basic friendliness of the people of both California and Scandinavia have not solved these problems.

Why Expensive Perfumes Don't Work

Studies by Alan Hirsch and Jason Gruss (Smell and Taste Treatment Research Foundation, Chicago and University of Michigan) found that expensive perfumes are much less effective than many essential oils and common foods. They studied the effects of several different scents on sexual arousal of males and females by comparing the subjects' blood flow in sexually aroused tissues (penile or clitoral blood flow) while wearing scented masks and while wearing nonodorized, blank masks. Expensive perfumes increased blood flow by only 3 percent in men. In contrast, the combined odor of lavender and pumpkin produced a 40 percent increase in men, and many other scents also worked better than the perfumes. While these results are for men, the researchers reported that women also responded poorly to expensive perfumes and positively to other smells. Hirsch suggests that certain scents may increase sexual arousal by acting on the brain in three different ways: by reducing anxiety, which inhibits natural sexual desire; increasing alertness and awareness, making the subjects more aware of sexual cues in the environment around them; and acting directly to the septal nuclei, a portion of the brain that induces sexual arousal.[4]

Effect of Perfumes and Scents on Blood Blow in Male Sexual Tissue:

Item Tested	Median % Increase in Penile Blood Flow
Lavender & Pumpkin Pie	40
Pumpkin Pie & Doughnut	20
Orange	19.5
Black Licorice & Cola	13
Black Licorice	3
Lily of the Valley	11
Vanilla	9
Pumpkin Pie	8.5
Lavender	8
Musk	7.5
Peppermint	6
Cheese Pizza	5
Roasting Meat	5
Rose	4
Strawberry	3.5
Oriental Spices	3.5
Expensive Perfumes	Averaged 3.0
Chocolate	2.8

Women: Effect of Perfumes & Scents on Enhancement of Clitoral Blood Flow

Item Tested	Median % Increase
Cucumber and Licorice Candy	13
Baby Powder	13
Lavender & Pumpkin Pie	11
Charcoal Barbecued Meat	Inhibited: Anti-arousal
Cherries	Inhibited: Anti-arousal
Expensive Men's Colognes	Inhibited: Anti-arousal

Above chart based on publications of Alan Hirsch and Jason Gruss[4]

Efforts to Create an Effective Perfume

Several companies have been set up to develop romantic pheromones, based on "the" putative human pheromone, for the general consumer, but most have had disappointing results.

For me, the use of aromatic plant oils as body perfumes was just an idea. Women who had been buying my experimental cosmetics with copper peptides kept asking me about perfumes, so I read everything that I could find. My conclusions were:

1. If pheromones are species-specific, humans shouldn't be able to detect animal-derived pheromones. But even if they could, what reactions might we expect? Taking into account that many animals become more dangerous during mating periods, humans shouldn't be attracted to the smell of a ready-to-mate boar; they should feel fear or aggression.

Androstenone triggers both sexual attraction and aggression in boars. In mice, certain pheromones cause male mice to kill other male mice (male odors increase attacks, female odors decrease attacks). Male lions and bears will kill the offspring of a female in order to mate with her. If purely sexual human pheromones, similar to pig androstenone, were discovered, they couldn't be used in perfume. If humans followed the urge for pheromone-induced mating, people would get arrested!

2. Human interactions are complex, and the social element is very important. There could be 100 human pheromones that affect different aspects of behavior.

3. Some musk-smelling plant pheromones, which are used by plants to attract bees and other pollinators to their flowers, are very similar to animal pheromones. Nature uses the same systems over and over again. For example, musk is a strong pheromone from musk deer, musk ducks, musky moles, muskrats, musk ox, and musk beetles. But similar pheromones exist in musk melons, musk hyacinths, musk cherries, musk thistle, musk rose, musk plums, and musk wood.

Elephants and some 140 species of moth share a similar female pheromone, but they don't get confused because for the moth, complementary chemicals must be present, and for the elephant, a signal from a moth is too minute.[5]

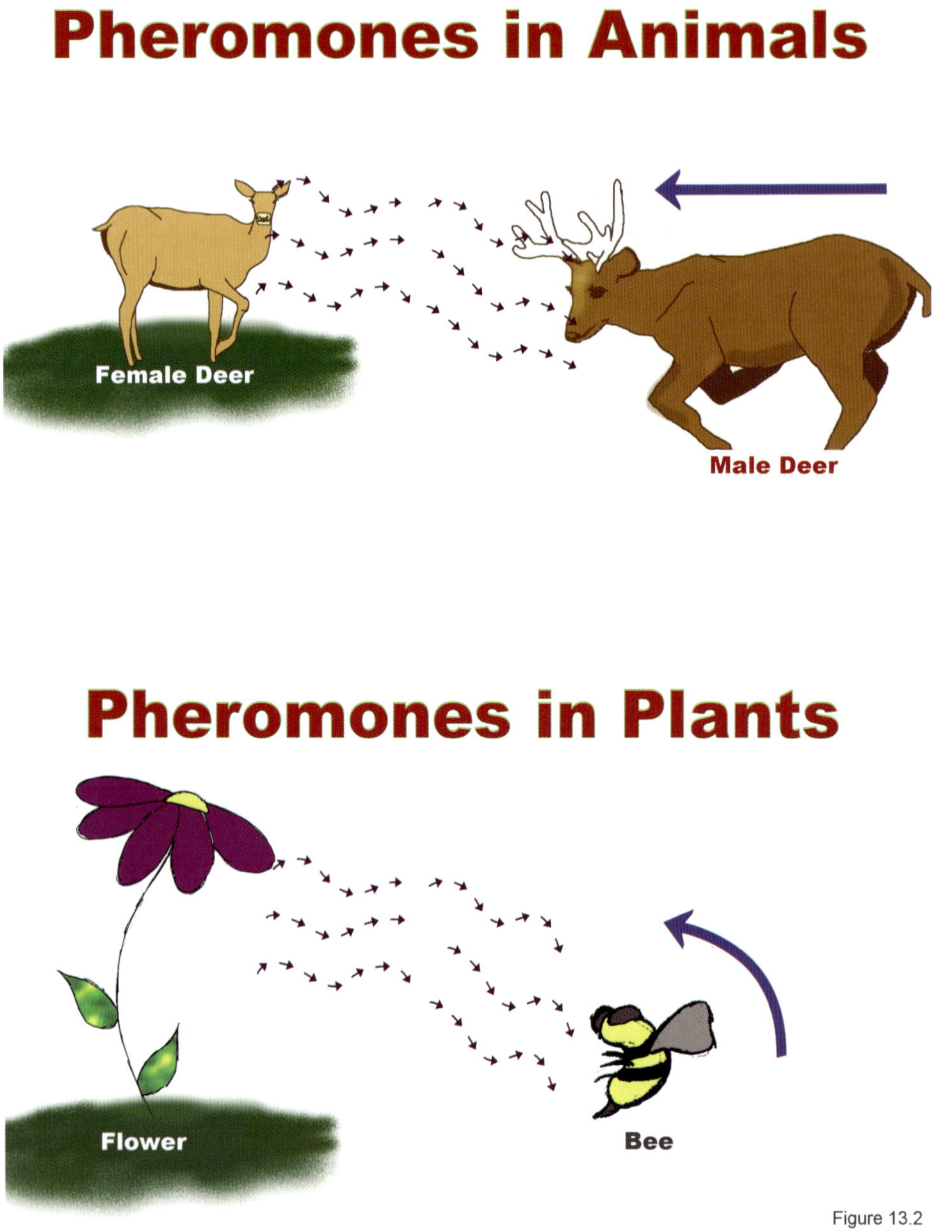

Pheromones in Animals

Female Deer

Male Deer

Pheromones in Plants

Flower

Bee

Figure 13.2

4. Dreaming of a pheromone perfume with aphrodisiac effects, the cosmetic industry doesn't take into account the importance of one's unique personal odor, which might be even more important in social bonding and sexual attraction.

5. Many pure essential oils have a long reputation as behavior modifiers. For example, in South Asia they are used in weddings, family gatherings, and religious ceremonies. Even the Bible speaks of women who have increased their beauty by applying scented oil. Such traditional oils have anti-conflict and harmonizing actions in both humans and animals.[6]

> *"Thy God hath anointed you with the oil of gladness."*
> – Saint Paul

6. When creating pheromone perfumes, most companies just use the molecule with the chemical smell rather than the original essential oil. But we don't know which component of the complex mixture is able to communicate with our brain, and it might even be an odorless component. By throwing away everything but the part that the nose can smell, these companies might also be throwing away the magic.

7. Historically, many of the traditional mood-altering essential oils have also been used for skin care. Patchouli has long been used as an anti-inflammatory and aid for dry, cracked skin. The oil of lavender has soothing effects on the skin and was applied to wounds in ancient Greece and Rome, and is still used today. Sandalwood is used for skin regeneration and to treat acne, dry skin, rashes, chapped skin, eczema, itching, and sensitive skin and also has anti-skin cancer actions. Ylang ylang is used to treat eczema, acne, oily skin, and irritation associated with insect stings or bites.[7]

With so many ways to benefit from essential oils, it is difficult to find a reason not to use them.

From Theory to Practice

At Skin Biology, for an experiment, I purchased a variety of very expensive human pheromones from other companies and gave them to volunteers for testing. I also gave the volunteers various pheromones from the essential oils of plants. The volunteers were asked to wear each of the pheromones and record people's reactions. Not surprisingly, in every case, the test subjects found few positive responses to the expensive human pheromones. Conversely, all of the volunteers reported positive responses to at least some of the tested plant pheromones, including people being more friendly, talkative, and affectionate. In these informal tests, based on client responses, I have found the most effective plant pheromones to be the essential oils of jasmine, ylang-ylang, nutmeg, sandalwood, Asian oud, patchouli, and lavender.

Body Perfumes with Plant Derived Pheromones

Based on our experiments, Skin Biology was able to create effective pheromone products that have won rave reviews from clients: Body Perfumes with Plant Derived Pheromones. There are several different scents to choose from, including patchouli (good for attracting women), ylang ylang (good for attracting men), musk, sandalwood, and jasmine (all universal attractants). A full list is available at www.SkinBiology.com. By using an appropriate version of Body Perfume on your body instead of regular perfume, you can strongly modify your personal "odor signature" in a positive way.

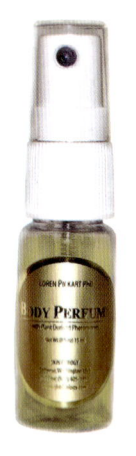

Think Torso and Legs, Not Wrists and Earlobes

For thousands of years, perfumes were applied to the torso and legs. The heat of the body would evaporate the pheromones and scents in the oil and blend them into a person's individual odor signature, a complex mixture of pheromones, body oils, fatty acids, sweat, and hormones such as androsterone secreted onto the skin from the apocrine glands. In addition, the 40 million skin cells that you shed each day add to your odor signature.

The modern method of applying perfumes to the wrists and earlobes only reflects the ignorance of the modern cosmetic industry. Body perfumes are best applied after a bath or shower. Dry yourself, and then spray on your body, especially on large, heat-producing areas such as the chest, breasts, and legs. If you bathe at night, the oils should be applied to your dry skin in the morning.

Finding the Body Perfume with Plant Derived Pheromone that best complements your unique odor signature and attracts the type of people that you desire may take some trial and error. Work your way through the oils one by one until you find the one that is most effective. Apply the oil, and then dress normally and go about your daily routine. If the oil is working, responsive people will unconsciously notice you from three to five feet away. Watch for people who unexpectedly turn and smile or extend conversations. Using plant-derived pheromones is a little like trolling for salmon using different lures; it takes some time, but keep trying and eventually you'll find the right lure (scent).

Client Testimonials:

Here's what some Skin Biology clients have to say about the Body Perfume with Plant Derived Pheromones.

"I've been using either the jasmine or the stealth version before company meetings with male executives. Now that I use the oil, they very often agree with me. Their aggression level seems to drop when I have Calypso's Oil on…I will just keep this method secret."
-Anonymous client from New York

"Whenever I use ylang ylang and nutmeg oil, I always get compliments, such as 'What are you wearing? I really have to know…"
-K.S.

"I am 60 years old, and the oil is working better than Viagra for me. I prefer the oils with ylang ylang and jasmine. My wife agrees."
-R.S.

"I love the stuff. I got the jasmine-scented one with the pheromones. It's not oily at all…a little goes a long way and soaks right in. I put it on my neck and shoulders, and not two minutes later my husband was kissing my neck."
-L.E.

"I tried the sample and was amazed at the number of people who either talked to me or told me how well I smelled."
-L.

"I tried the ylang ylang, nutmeg, and SB-74. I rubbed the oil on my upper body and breasts in the morning, and then went about my usual day. I was amazed at the number of men who started friendly conversations with me. It's great!"
-F.H.

"I would just like to add another affirmation of these Body Perfumes. They are definitely winners. I've been wearing them since my last order a few months back, and I can assuredly say that they are quite addictive. They kind of have a bit of an aromatherapeutic lift for me in addition to their powers of attraction…Great job, Skin Biology!"
-K.

Plant-Derived Pheromones

(Note: These are general comments from our clients. Responses may vary widely among individuals.)

Mood Enhancer	Mood Effects	Effects on Women	Effects on Men	Traditional Uses
Lavender	Calming Relaxing Soothing	YES	YES	Skin healing, beneficial for acne, burns, wounds, rashes, psoriasis, PMS, stress, tension, and muscle cramps.
Jasmine	Erotic Very Pleasant	STRONG	MODERATE	Aphrodisiac: Said to increase arousal, attractiveness, seductiveness, and appeal. Emotionally produces feelings of optimism, confidence, euphoria, reduces tension, anxiety and depression, relieves menstrual cramps and pain.
Asian Oud	Calming Erotic	STRONG	STRONG	A historical favorite in Arab countries, produced by a fungus that lives on trees.
Ylang Ylang	Erotic Relaxing	MODERATE	STRONG	Strong aphrodisiac: said to increase arousal and attachment. Traditionally spread on the marriage bed in Bali.
Sandalwood	Erotic, Musk-like, Relaxing	MODERATE	STRONG	Scent is very similar to musks from animals such as deer musk, civitone musk from civit cats, and castorium from beavers which are traditional aphrodisiacs for both men and women.
Nutmeg	Energizing	STRONG	STRONG	Very stimulating, helps with frigidity, impotence, neuralgia, and nervous fatigue. Used for better circulation, arthritis, gout, muscular aches and pains.
Patchouli	Mildly Erotic	STRONG	LOW	A favorite of women: erotic for women, probably not on men.

Chapter 14

Glowing Good Health:

Better Suntanning with Less Skin Damage

Magazines and the TV news are filled with stories about the dangers of tanning your skin. As a result, you probably apply sunscreen, or at least wear a wide-brimmed hat, whenever you are in the sun for even a short period of time. But is it really healthy to avoid the sun? Consider the following: Humans evolved in the presence of abundant sunlight. Geneticists and archaeologists calculate that our ancestors lost their body hair 1.2 million years ago but only started wearing clothes 72,000 years ago. So for more than 1,128,000 years, our forebearers lived in splendid nudity and thrived. The following is additional evidence that human skin thrives when exposed to sunlight.[1]

— In the United States, people in professions with high sunlight exposure (such as farmers and mail carriers) live the longest.
— Cancer rates are highest in the northern states with the least sunshine.
— Rates of the major cancers are drastically lower in persons with more sunlight exposure.
— Sunlight-associated cancers increased most in the places where sunscreen was most heavily promoted.
— Sunlight improves the moods of persons with seasonal affective disorder.
— Psoriatic skin lesions are reduced by sunlight.
— Sunlight raises testosterone levels in males.
— Sunlight exposure may reduce the incidence of schizophrenia.
— Multiple sclerosis is lowest in the areas with the most sunlight.
— Sunlight improves bone health.
— Sunlight decreases auto-immune diseases such as multiple sclerosis, Type 1 diabetes, and rheumatoid arthritis.

Figure 14.1

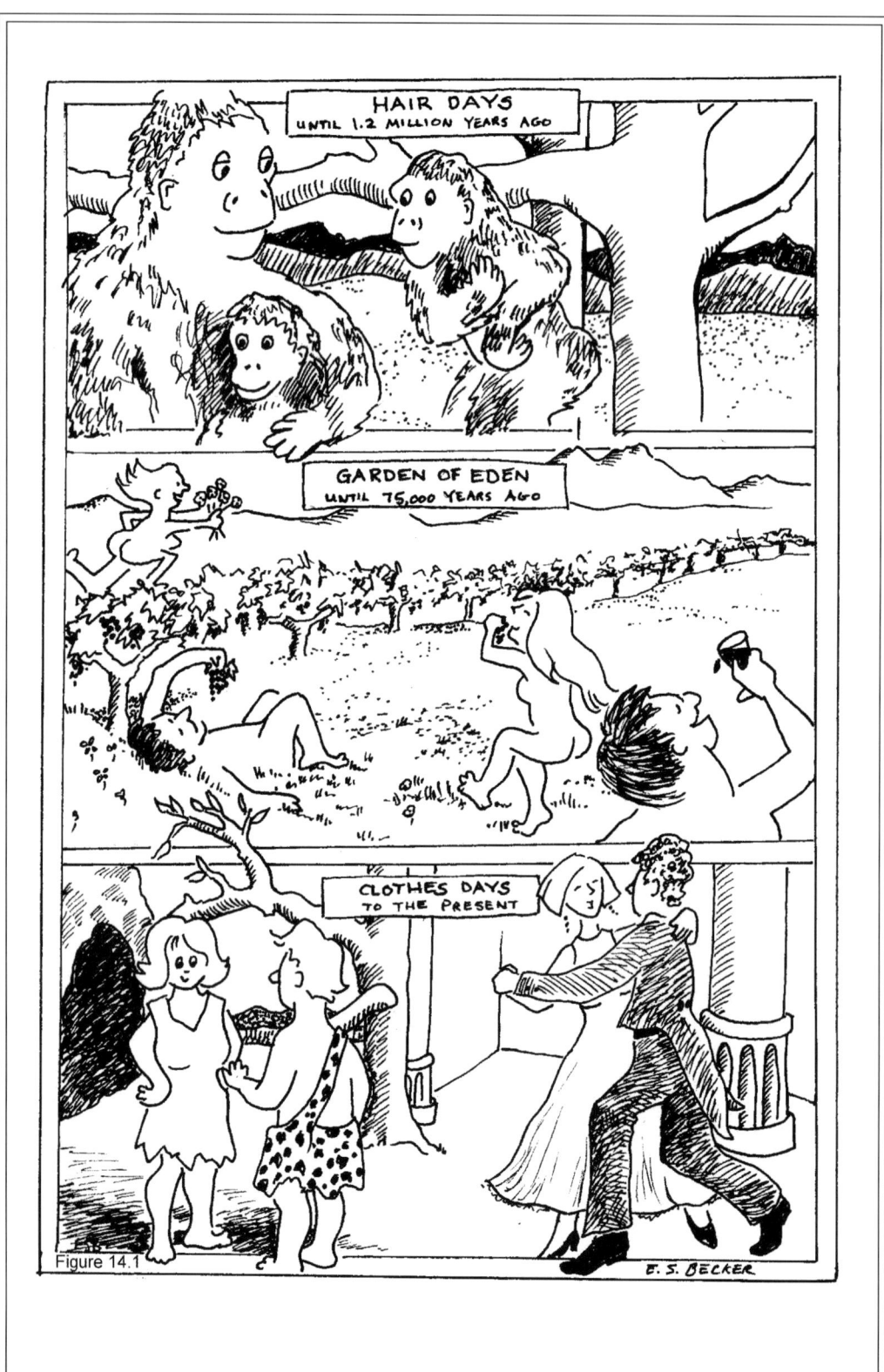

Sunlight and Good Health

A certain amount of sunlight on your skin is necessary for good health. Sunlight activates a gene called pom-C that in turn helps create melanin, which determines skin color and also enhances sex drive (the endorphins or "happiness hormones"), as well as leptin, which helps burn fat and keep you thin. Sunlight also produces vitamin D in the skin and strongly affects the brain's pineal gland function, which controls many bodily functions. While positive actions of sunlight are often attributed to an increased production of vitamin D, the cause is likely to be more complex. Sunlight generates many other molecules in the skin, perhaps dozens or hundreds more. Still waiting in the shadows are more discoveries on skin biochemistry than are dreamt of in dermatology.

While sunlight is necessary for good health, the ultraviolet (UV) rays in sunlight do cause skin damage. The question is how to find methods of receiving adequate sunlight exposure while reducing skin damage.[1-2]

Sensible Suntanning

The idea of a sensible suntan probably sounds like an oxymoron if you have spent years avoiding the sun, but it is possible. The goal is to increase your skin's melanin production while minimizing damage. A build-up of melanin helps block UV rays and also serves as a free radical scavenger.

The key to sensible suntanning is to tan slowly. For most people, suntanning for a maximum of 20 to 30 minutes a day produces the best results. One exception is those afflicted with seasonal affective disorder, who often need several hours of full-spectrum lighting a day to alleviate depression. Whole-body suntanning is the most efficient and safest method since the large skin area permits maximum sunlight exposure in the shortest amount of time. On the other hand, children generally need less sun than adults; most have thin skin that burns quickly and should not be exposed to sunlight for more than five to 10 minutes at a time. Infants under age 1 should be protected from intense sunlight at all times.

When you tan sensibly, your skin's natural protective system is able to defend you. This protective system includes defenses against oxygen radicals, such as vitamin E and beta-carotene, as well as copper-zinc superoxide dismutase, which detoxifies oxygen radicals and reduces skin damage.

Another aspect of sensible suntanning, besides monitoring how much sun you get, is to follow a protective regimen on tropical vacations and other occasions when you will be exposed to the sun. The following are a few steps I recommend:

OLD-FASHIONED SUNSCREENS

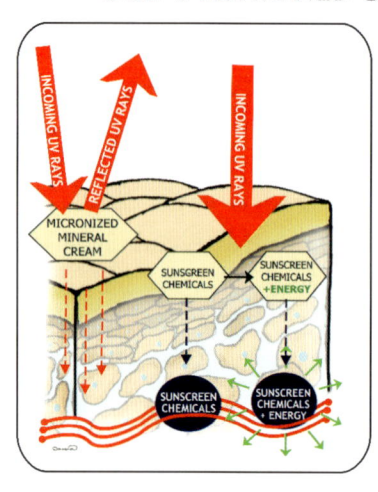

SUN SCREENS with MICRONIZED MINERALS

Can penetrate and Accumulate in lower Layer of Skin

UV ABSORBING SUNSCREEN CHEMICALS:

As much as 35% of Sunscreen Chemicals enter the blood stream

SUNSCREEN CHEMICALS + ENERGY:

Once sunscreen chemicals Combine with Energy they can Enter the blood stream and Damage the DNA

HEALTHIER SUN PROTECTION

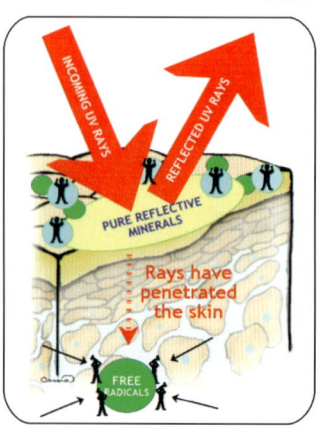

PROTECTIVE CREAM on SKIN
ANTIOXIDANTS & Pure Reflective Minerals
Topically protect skin from Free Radical formation:

SRCPs
Vitamin E Family
Tocotrienol Family
CoQ10
Lycopene
Leutin

🕴 = PROTECT

🕴 = BREAK DOWN

PROTECTIVE ANTIOXIDANTS within SKIN
Fight off Free Radical formation:

Superoxide Dismutase
Vitamin E Family
Tocotrienol Family
CoQ10
Lycopene
Leutin
Vitamin C

🟢 = FREE RADICALS

🟡 = PURE REFLECTIVE MINERALS

🔵 = ANTIOXIDANTS

Figure 14.2

© Loren Pickart PhD

1. Prior to suntanning, apply a thin coat of Skin Biology's Protect & Restore Suntanning Lotion. This is a skin remodeling cream with titanium dioxide and high levels of antioxidants. A small amount of water may be used to help spread the cream.

2. After suntanning, apply Protect & Restore Body Lotion. Suntanning produces damage to the skin barrier that must be promptly repaired to reduce peeling. Skin Biology's SRCP creams help the process of skin barrier repair.

3. If you have a tendency to burn or plan to spend an extended amount of time in the sun, use a reflective sunscreen, such as titanium dioxide, over the Protect & Restore Suntanning Lotion.

4. Three days prior to tanning, take a daily supplement of vitamin C (1 g), Co-Q10 (30 mgs), alpha lipoic acid (100 mgs), vitamin E (400 units), and tocotrienols (35 mgs). Other skin researchers have recommended daily beta carotene (30 mg), mixed carotenoids from algae (50 mg), Vitamin E (400 units), and Vitamin C (1 g).

5. Sunglasses that absorb UV rays should be worn for eye protection. Large hats and protective clothing should be worn during times of prolonged sunlight exposure.

6. Sunlight over your entire body, such as being nude (as our ancestors were for a million years) or in a bathing suit, produces maximum sunlight benefits with minimum skin damage.

But for how long should you expose your nude (or swim suited) body to sunlight in a day? Here are some old answers. Sunlight was used as a medicine for thousands of years. A century ago, there were many clinics in European mountain regions where whole body sunlight treatments were used on patients with skin wounds and infections. The prescribed sunlight exposure was 15 to 30 minutes twice daily. Physicians were warned not to start sunlight exposure too rapidly.

Too Much of a Good Thing

While a moderate amount of sun exposure is beneficial, too much sun can overwhelm the skin's protective system. Lester Packer (University of California, Berkeley) found that as UV radiation dosage is increased, the skin's antioxidant defenses are overwhelmed, allowing free radicals to form and cause cellular damage, such as lipid peroxidation and oxidative modification of proteins and cellular DNA. As little as 45 minutes of exposure to the noon-day sun can reduce the skin's protective vitamin C

> "L'assaut au soleil
> des blancheurs des corps de femme...
> (The assault on the sunlight
> by the whiteness of women's bodies...)"
> — Arthur Rimbaud 1854-1891

levels by 80 percent and lower other skin antioxidants. It takes the melanocytes in the skin two to fives days to produce protective melanin. In contrast, a severe burn can occur in just a few hours.[3]

The bottom line is: You can't rush a sensible suntan. Development of a healthy tan takes a minimum of one to two weeks. As your body is exposed to the sun, a thickening of the skin occurs, which increases your resistance to burning.

Be careful about sun exposure if you take medication such as tetracycline, antihistamines, "sulfa" drugs, diuretics, and some oral contraceptives as these medications can make your skin more sensitive to light.

Pure Reflective Sunblockers

If you plan to spend hours basking on the beach and want protection from the sun, use a pure reflective sunblocker. These products contain inert minerals such as titanium dioxide, zinc oxide, red petrolatum, and talc and work by reflecting (rather than absorbing) UV rays.

Choose a pure reflective sunblocker with an appropriate sun protection factor (SPF) based on how much time you plan to spend in the sun. An SPF of 15 will provide 15 times the amount of protection you'd get without using anything. So if 10 minutes in the sun is enough to turn you red, a sunscreen with an SPF of 15 would allow you to stay out for 150 minutes before burning.

The best reflective sunblockers are pure titanium dioxide and zinc oxide. These minerals are usually white in color and are difficult to formulate into a transparent product. But pasty, white coloring is the price of sun protection. Avoid micronized minerals that are coated with silicone or other chemicals to make them transparent because the coated mineral penetrates deeply into the lower skin layers.

Some feel that heavy use of zinc oxide increases facial pore size. If skin acids release ionic zinc from zinc oxide, this may enter the skin and inhibit the skin repair actions of ionic copper.

Chemical Sunscreens Aren't the Answer

You might be tempted to reach for any old bottle of sunscreen on the grocery store shelf to protect yourself from the sun. Don't. Chemical sunscreens contain oily chemicals that strongly absorb the energy in light photons and can cause more harm than good.

Many dermatologists advocate that chemical sunscreens applied before exposure to sunlight prevent skin cancer. Yet epidemiological studies have failed to find an anti-cancer action of sunscreen. In 1998, epidemiologist Marianne Berwick of the Sloan-Kettering Cancer Center analyzed 16 studies of sunscreen use, with mixed results. She reported that four studies suggested sunscreen protects against skin cancer; five studies found no effect; and seven studies found a higher rate of cancer with sunscreen use. Her conclusion was that "Sunscreen may not protect against skin cancer" and "We don't really know whether sunscreen prevents skin cancer."[4]

In the opinion of ultra-marathoner Dr. Gordon Ainsleigh, sunscreen use might actually increase the number of cancer deaths. After analyzing a 17 percent rise in the breast cancer rate, he stated that the increase could be the result of sunscreen use. Dr. Ainsleigh also concluded that there are 2,200 sunlight-associated cancer deaths annually in the U.S., versus 138,000 for sunlight-inhibited cancers. Worldwide, the greatest rise in melanoma has occurred in Queensland, Australia, where sunscreen use is heavily promoted. Most Australians grew up hearing the slogan "Slip, Slap, Slop" with regard to sunscreen. In other words, they were told the more sunscreen they used, the better.[5]

Is ozone depletion, rather than sunscreen, the culprit? Not likely. Johan Moan of the Norwegian Cancer Institute found that from 1957 to 1984, the annual incidence of melanoma in Norway in men and women had increased by 350 percent and 440 percent respectively, but concluded that "ozone depletion is not the cause of the increase in skin cancer."[6]

Sunscreen Chemicals Have Three Primary Defects

They are powerful free radical generators	Their free radical generation increases cellular damage and changes that lead to cancer
They often have strong estrogenic activity	They increase risk of cancer and other medical problems
They are synthetic chemicals that are alien to the human body and accumulate in body fat stores	The human body is well adapted to detoxify biologicals that it has been exposed to over tens of millions of years. But it has often has difficulty removing non-biological compounds such as DDT, Dioxin, PCBs and chemical sunscreens

Why Sunscreen is Potentially Harmful

As an example of how damaging sunscreen chemicals can be, consider psoralen, a chemical used with UV light to treat psoriasis. Psoralen is similar to sunscreen chemicals, and the rate of skin cancer in patients treated with psoralen is 83 times higher than among the general population.[7]

Many sunscreen chemicals also have strong estrogenic (estrogen-like) actions that may cause problems in sexual development and adult sexual function. These include an increased rate of cancer, an increased rate of birth defects in children, a lower sperm count and smaller penis size in men, and a plethora of other medical problems. The effects are similar to those of many banned chemicals, such as DDT, dioxin, and PCBs.

Margaret Schlumpf and her colleagues (Institute of Pharmacology and Toxicology, Univ. of Zurich, Switzerland) have found that many widely used sunscreen chemicals mimic the effects of estrogen and trigger developmental abnormalities in rats.[8]

Expected Effects of Estrogenic Chemicals in Humans

In Women	
	Endometriosis
	Migraines
	Severe PMS
	Erratic Periods
	Increases in Breast and Uterine Cancer
	Fibrocystic Breast Disease
	Uterine Cysts
In Men	Lowered Sperm Count
	Breast Enlargement
	Smaller Than Normal Penis Size
	More Testicular Cancer
	Undescended Testicles
	Loss of Libido

> "Estrogenic sunscreen chemicals might explain most of the social changes in California over the past 30 years."
> — A California customer

Chapter 15

Feeding your Face and Body Nutrients that Turn Back the Clock

Human aging has many causes, including genetic developmental programs, adequacy of stem cell production for tissue repair and replacement, accumulation of oxidative damage, and changes in the amount of key biochemical compounds, and growth factors. But by eating a diet rich in fruits, vegetables, and other nutritionally valuable foods and taking the proper supplements, you can slow, and in some cases even reverse, the hands of time. That's right! By eating a nutrient rich diet, we not only turn back the hands of time, we nourish our skin as well . . . so those hands of time appear smooth and wrinkle free.

During aging, many critical biochemical substances, such as DHEA and alpha lipoic acid, decline sharply. As a result, the biochemical balances that produced a youthful body are lost and aging accelerates. The goal of diet changes and supplements is to restore the biochemical balances that once produced a young, healthy body. We are what we eat and so is our skin.

The process is similar to the problem that existed 80 years ago for individuals with juvenile diabetes caused by a lack of insulin. Today the biochemical lack of insulin, which once led to an early death, is effectively treated by supplemental insulin and people with juvenile diabetes can live a normal lifespan.

Eating right and enhancing your diet with supplements benefits your health in many ways. These include increasing your antioxidant defenses and restoring the critical biochemicals that decline with age. Certain supplements also improve your skin and hair. For example, methylsulfonylmethane (MSM) has long been used to speed hair growth in horses, and vitamin C is needed for collagen contraction and skin tightening.

50,000 Years of Dietary Changes

Despite advances in research on nutrition, there is still much debate over what foods make up the optimal diet. Perhaps the best approach is to consider how human nutrition has evolved since our ancestor's time.

The anatomy of the human body suggests that we are designed to eat a diet consisting of many different food sources. Pure plant-eaters, such as cattle and horses, have large intestines designed for the extraction of energy from grasses and leaves; while pure carnivores, such as lions and wolves, have short intestines that extract nutrients from easily digestible meats. But humans have an extended intestine, though much smaller than that of an herbivore, that is able to digest both plants and meats.

The primary source of human nutrition has fluctuated throughout history. Humans descended from plant-eating primates that subsisted on a diet consisting mainly of plant sources (97 percent), especially fruits, vegetables, nuts, and roots. Then, about 50,000 years ago, greatly improved hunting and fishing abilities prompted a radical transformation in the human diet, to a diet high in protein and fat. A second major change came about 10,000 years ago, when grains were cultivated by early hunter-farmers. A new grain-heavy diet was born, which included high-calorie meats but cut out a large portion of the plant fiber that had previously been consumed.

A final change came within the last 400 years, when the consumption of sugar dramatically increased, from about two pounds a year during the Stone Age to about 130 pounds a year (in the U.S.). In addition, alcoholic beverages became more readily available, and alcohol consumption increased by a factor of 10 to 20-fold.

Today, the foods we eat are often altered from their natural forms. One of the most damaging examples of processed food is trans-fats, fats that have been hardened by chemical hydrogenation, which solidifies liquid vegetable oil into hard fats such as shortening and margarine. Frequently found in French fries, doughnuts, cookies, pastries, crackers, and many other processed foods, trans-fats have been shown to increase the incidence of cardiovascular disease, diabetes, obesity, cataracts, arthritis, and cancer.

The amount and types of fat many humans eat reinforces how much our diet has changed over the centuries. Among the essential fatty acids (EFAs), or fatty acids required for normal human growth and development that must come from our diet, are two families which serve as starting materials for many of the body's hormones and other regulatory molecules: omega-3s (present in fish oils) and omega-6s (found in plant oils). Early humans consumed a diet that was approximately equal in both of these classes of fats. Today, people in the U.S. eat about 14 times more omega-6 than omega-3 EFAs. This imbalance negatively impacts the production of many of our critical regulatory molecules and makes us more prone to inflammatory and cardiovascular diseases.

The modern diet has other negative effects as well. Tooth decay was minimal before the easy availability of simple sugars, and many medical historians insist that modern heart disease only developed after approximately 1850. Ancient medical writings from China, Europe, and the Middle East, going back over 2,500 years, do not describe the characteristic symptoms of a modern heart attack, although the same ancient writings describe many other modern diseases.

Dietary Changes from the Stone Age:

	Stone Age	Present Day Americans	Effect of Change
Simple Sugars	2 lbs. / year	130 lbs. / year	Diabetes, tooth decay
Essential Fatty Acids	Omega-6 is about equal to Omega-3	About 14 times more Omega-6 than Omega-3	More cancer, blood clots, auto-immune disease, depression
Trans-fats Hydrogenated Fats	Very little	High in processed foods	Damage to cell membranes, more cancer and immunological diseases
Minerals	High in mountain areas with long lifespan	Lower because of processed foods	More heart disease, cancer, and arthritis
Meat	Hunted animals were low in fat: 3% fat	Farmed animals high in fat	Heart disease, diabetes, obesity
Soluble Fiber	High vegetable fiber diet	Low fiber diet	Intestinal problems

GENERAL DIETARY CHANGES

Nature's Medicine: Fruits and Vegetables

Our body needs about 40 essential nutrients that it cannot synthesize and many of these are obtained from plants. A balanced, unprocessed diet rich in fruits and vegetables provides our bodies with the vitamins and minerals they need to thrive, as well as valuable phytonutrients and antioxidants. The most fundamental change in the human diet over the centuries has been the sharp reduction in the intake of low-calorie plant foods. Our bodies are still designed for a diet high in fruits and vegetables, such as cabbage, apples, lettuce, berries, and so forth.

The common fruits and vegetables sold at your neighborhood grocery store are as powerful as any preventative medicine available at the pharmacy. These unprocessed plant foods contain a wide variety of more than 600 phytonutrients that benefit our health, including terpenes, organosulfides, isothiocyanates, indoles, dithiolthiones, polyphenols, flavones, tannins, and protease inhibitors.

Fruits and vegetables also contain carotenoids, a rich source of vitamin A and antioxidants. The carotenoids lutein (abundant in spinach and other green leafy vegetables) and lycopene (found in tomatoes) possess particularly strong antioxidant activity. This is important because as we age, our antioxidant defenses decline and must be enhanced to reduce free radical damage. Free radicals cause damage responsible for degenerative diseases such as arthritis, heart disease, cancer, and senility. Examples are in the following charts:

Level of Oxidative Damage with Age

Antioxidant Superoxide Dismutase Activity with Age

Antioxidant Melatonin with Age

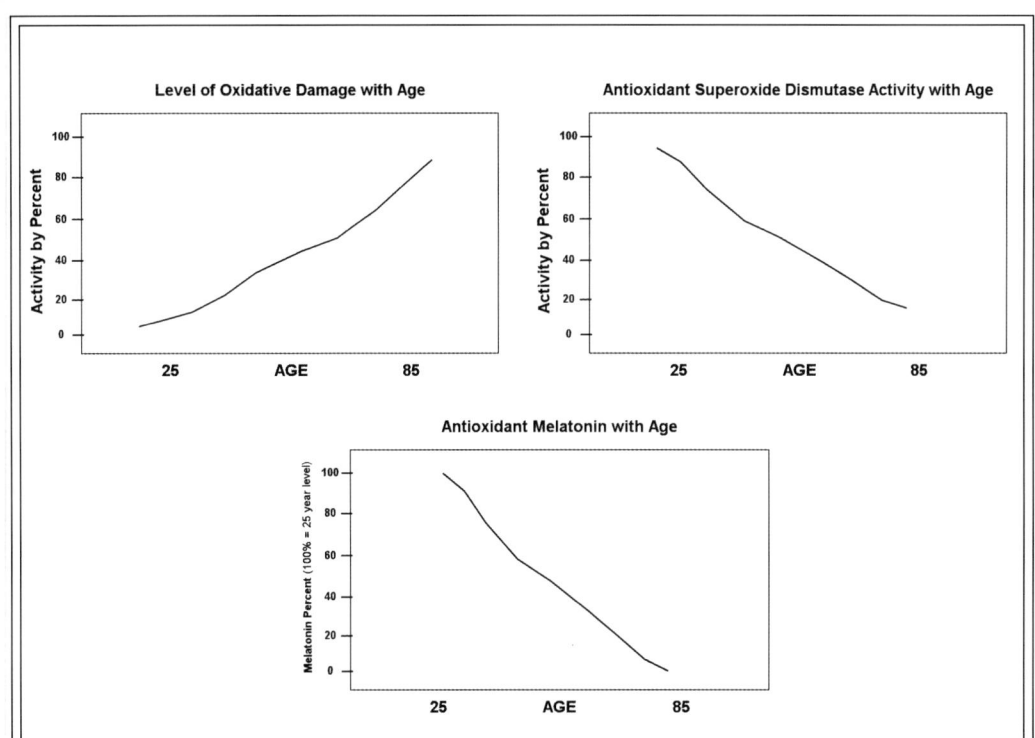

Charts Based on: Linnane A.W. et al [1]

Fruits and Vegetables are Powerful Antioxidants:

Decrease in Damaging Oxidations of Body Fats

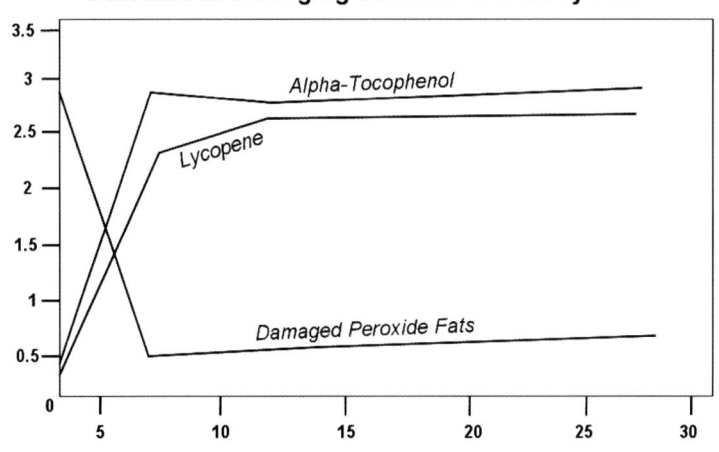

Days on Supplementation with Dehydrated Fruit and Vegetable Powders

Decrease in Damaging Oxidations of Body Fats (Based on: Wise et al)[2]

Antioxidants Need Not Be Expensive

Wise and colleagues reported that the daily supplement of 1.5 grams of dried extracts of fruits and vegetables reduced damaging lipid peroxidation products in the blood by 75 percent within one week. Lipid peroxidation products are an excellent measure of the rate of damaging oxidations within the body. Conversely, protective antioxidants such as alpha-tocopherol and lycopene sharply rose. The fruit and vegetable supplements consisted of dried fruit and vegetable powders obtained by drying juices from apples, oranges, pineapples, papaya, cranberries, peaches, carrots, parsley, beets, broccoli, kale, cabbage, spinach, and tomatoes.[2]

Fresh vs. Processed Juice

Many people get a regular dose of fruits and vegetables through drinking juice. But some juices might be better for us than others. While processed juice has many health benefits, some nutritionists say that freshly prepared juice is healthier. Fresh juice contains a significant level of hydrogen peroxide, which some scientists say serves as a natural stimulant to the immune system. Human mothers milk also contains a significant level of hydrogen peroxide. Unfortunately, the amount of hydrogen peroxide in juice drops rapidly during storage.

Sugars and Carbohydrates

Simple sugars should be drastically limited. But be aware that FDA regulations only consider sucrose as sugar. Non-sugar foods may contain fructose, glucose, high fructose corn syrup and maltose, fruit juice concentrates, honey, dextrose, lactose, maltose, and molasses, all of which are sugars that are no better than sucrose. Whole fruits, vegetables and unprocessed grains provide essential sugars from complex carbohydrates without affecting blood sugar levels and increasing the need for insulin. But processed carbohydrates such as white bread, cake, potatoes and pasta are quickly broken down and raise blood sugar levels.[3]

Dietary Fiber

Another benefit of plant foods is that they are rich in dietary fiber. Most Americans don't eat nearly enough fiber; some nutritionists recommend that we consume 40 to 50 grams a day, but the average American gets only 12. There are two types of dietary fiber, insoluble and soluble, each of which has different sources and benefits. Insoluble fiber improves digestion and is predominant in plant skins, husks, and the tough part of plants. Soluble fiber helps reduce blood cholesterol and the risk of coronary artery disease and is found in pectin, guar, barley, and oat bran. You can increase your intake of both insoluble and soluble fiber by eating more whole-grain foods and cereal products, fruits, and vegetables.

Not Vitamins, but Vitamin Families

Vitamins are natural substances necessary in small amounts in the diet for the normal growth and maintenance of our bodies. Each of the six main vitamins (A, B, C, D, E and K) has its own vitamin family. For example, the vitamin C family consists of at least seven forms of vitamin C, while vitamin E has four forms plus its closely associated tocotrienol cousins. Vitamin A and beta-carotene are part of a family of at least 400 members. According to recent research, mixtures of vitamins may be better than the use of a pure vitamin.

Is the Recommended Daily Allowance Enough?

The Recommended Daily Allowance (RDA) is the list on processed foods and vitamin products that tells what percentage of each of 19 essential nutrients you get per serving or dose. However, what most people don't realize is that the RDA was not developed for humans, but rather is the minimum amount of daily nutrients needed for young rats to successfully breed. It doesn't take into account the changing nutritional needs of aging humans and persons with special diseases, such as diabetes and heart disease.

Much-needed changes to the RDA are slowly taking place. For example, the importance of a higher folic acid intake to reduce birth defects and heart disease has resulted in an increased RDA of folic acid. But keep in mind that the RDA is a flawed guide, especially as you get older. The following chart provides levels of some supplements recommended by experts on human aging to produce noticeable actions in the body. You may need only a few of these supplements depending on your personal health. For example, a person with cardiovascular disease may benefit more from omega-3 fats than the average person. However keep in mind that supplements do not substitute for good quality foods that contain a wide range of helpful nutrients, some of which science is not yet aware of. Our bodies are complex and so are the nutrients in foods we consume. It's all a balancing act to find what works best for yourself.

Supplements & Vitamins Recommended by Many Anti-Aging Scientists

This information is to illustrate important supplements used to restore internal biochemical balances.
You may not need all these supplements. (g=gram, mg=milligram)

	Vitamins & Supplements	Recommended per Day	Principal Action
Protective Antioxidants	Alpha Lipoic Acid	30-200 mg	Master Antioxidant
	Vitamin C	0.5 to 1 gram	
	Coenzyme Q-10	30-200 mg	
	Vitamin E family (all isomers)	400 mg	
	Tocotrienols family	35-75 mg	
	Lutein	20 mg	
	Lycopene	5 mg	
	Grape Seed Extract	50 mg	
	Vegetable Extracts	1000-2000 mg	Mixture of antioxidants
	Melatonin	1-3 mg at bedtime	Helps sleep, protects brain
Essential Oils	Omega-3 Oils	1-5 grams Salmon/Flaxseed/Canola oil	See chapter text
	Omega-6 Oil Gamma Linolenic Acid	1-3 grams Borage Oil	Anti-inflammatory omega-6 fat helps skin integrity, joint lubrication
Brain and Nerves	Ginkgo Biloba	60 mg	
	N-acetyl-carnitine	0.5 to 1 gram	
	Choline/Inositol	1-2 grams	
Minerals	Calcium	1-2 grams	
	Magnesium	500 mg	
	Zinc	7-15 mg	
	Copper	2-4 mg	
Hair	Saw Palmetto Oil	80-160 mg	Reduces DHT
	Soy Flavones		Estrogen effects
Elements of Collagen and Extra-cellular Matrix Proteins	MSM	0.5 to 1 gram	For joints and hair
	Vitamin C	500-1000 mg	For collagen
	Glucosamine	0.5 to 1.5 grams	For skin extracellular matrix and joints
	Chondroitin Sulfate	0.4 to 1.2 grams	For skin extracellular matrix and joints
NITROGEN OXIDE RELEASERS	Arginine/Ornithine	1-2 grams	Vasodilator
EXTRA SOLUBLE FIBER		5-20 grams	
Red Wine		5-15 oz.	Increases happiness, reduces illness
Folic Acid		400 mg	Reduces illness
DHEA		25-100 mg	Increases sexual and metabolic hormones and blocks cortisone damage

Not All Fat Is Bad for You

As mentioned previously, EFAs are fatty acids that are necessary for good health. They fall into two families: omega-3 and omega-6, which differ only in the number and placement of the double bonds on their carbon chains. Some researchers recommend getting at least 3 percent of daily calories from EFAs. Because the present U.S. diet has much more omega-6 fats than omega-3 fats, increasing your omega-3 fats is most important.

There are different types of omega-3 fats, which are required in different amounts. For eicosapentaenoic acid (EPA) and docosahexanoic acid (DHA), some experts recommend an intake of 300 to 400 mg per day. Taking omega-3 supplements can help you meet your daily requirement while avoiding the problem of mercury that is found in some ocean fish. These types of omega-3s are found primarily in oily cold-water fish such as tuna, salmon, and mackerel. Fish oils, the best source of the omega-3 fats, are easiest taken in the Enteric Coated Capsule form that does not have the fishy taste or smell and is only released when the capsule reaches the intestines. Plant oils such as flaxseed and canola oil also contain omega-3 fats, but in lower concentrations.

One more essential fat, gamma linolenic acid, is produced in the body but declines sharply with age. Although this is an omega-6 fat, it has anti-inflammatory actions, improves skin integrity, and aids joint lubrication. Borage oil, 1 to 3 grams daily, is the best source of this fat.

Limit Calories

Many researchers on human aging say that eating less and limiting total calorie intake, especially as one becomes older, can improve health. Humans evolved in a world of daily food gathering that was not always successful and short periods of involuntary fasting were common.

Using the Right Fat: The Lyon Heart Diet

As far as the medical community is concerned, olive oil is the best oil for cooking. A diet rich in olive oil reduces the risk of stroke and breast cancer. For every 1 percent increase in the intake of monounsaturated fat, there is an 11 percent decrease in the risk of stroke.[4]

The benefits of olive oil were recently evidenced in The Lyon Heart Diet study, a trial designed to see if the typical Mediterranean diet is more protective than the much-touted low-fat, low-cholesterol diet. The Lyon Heart Diet is relatively high in fat, with the main sources of fat being olive oil and seafood. In the trial, more than 600 patients who had recovered from a first heart attack were randomly selected to either continue their present diet or start eating The Lyon Heart Diet. The Lyon Heart dieters were instructed to eat more fish, vegetables, and fruits; replace processed breads with real bread (e.g., traditional French bread); eat less meat and replace red meat with chicken; and use olive oil and canola oil as their sources of cooking fat.

Although The Lyon Heart Diet didn't reduce blood lipids, there was a 70 percent reduction in cardiac deaths and coronary events within one year (rising to a 76 percent reduction after two years), which correlated with the omega-3 content of the diet. After four years, there was also a 61 percent reduction in the risk of cancer, which may be due to anti-cancer actions of oleic acid. Blood samples taken from the patients found that the diet increased blood antioxidants (vitamins E and C) and omega-3 fats while reducing omega-6 fats. Surprisingly, there was no change in blood pressure or cholesterol with The Lyon Heart Diet in comparison to the control (normal diet) patients. The conclusion was that Mediterranean-style diets are one of the healthiest diets a person can eat.[5]

Red Wine and Your Health

Numerous studies have demonstrated that drinking one to two glasses of wine or beer daily results in an improvement in health. Red wine is thought to be the most effective.

The health-enhancing effect of red wine is hardly a new phenomenon, as the case of Luigi Cornaro shows. Luigi, a Venetian nobleman of the 16th century, discovered he was dying at age 40. He went on a daily diet of 12 ounces of bread, broth, and eggs, as well as 14 ounces of wine. Incredibly, Luigi Cornaro lived to see the ripe old age of 102.[6]

Moderate wine consumption may even improve our mental abilities. One study of 733 men and 1,053 women ages 55 to 88 found that men who drank four to six drinks and women who drank two to four drinks a day showed superior performance in many cognitive domains relative to abstainers.[7]

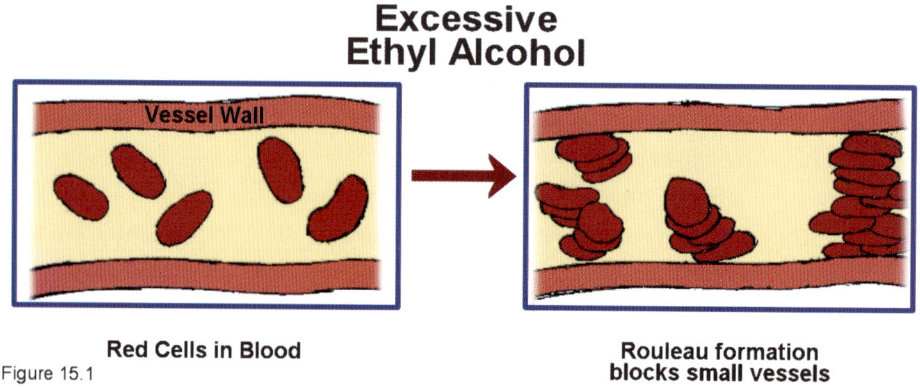

Excessive Ethyl Alcohol

Red Cells in Blood

Figure 15.1

Rouleau formation blocks small vessels

It should be noted that beyond two or three drinks a day, other factors, such as accidents, can become a health issue. In addition, heavy alcohol intake can generate levels of free radicals that overwhelm the liver's antioxidant defenses and produce damage. Rapid intake of alcohol can produce blood sludging in the smaller vessels due to rouleau formation as red blood cells bind to each other and form stacks of cells. This stops oxygen and nutrient flow to the affected tissues and can produce a rupture of the blood vessels.

Now let me personally make a toast to your healthy skin, heart, body, mind and senses. Eat and be well. Bon Appetite!

Chapter 16

The Science Behind SRCPs

SRCPs, the magic molecules to which much of this book is dedicated, arose from four decades of work by myself and colleagues in more than 40 research laboratories. As the name Skin Remodeling Copper Peptides implies, SRCPs refer to the skin, but the same molecule also activates the repair and remodeling of other tissues in the body, such as the hair follicles, stomach lining, intestinal tract, bones, and liver.

The path that led me to pursue a career in medical research, and later to the study of SRCPs, began in the Minnesota heartland where I grew up. When I was 10 years old, I caught a throat infection that had me in bed for two weeks. Then the doctor gave me a shot of penicillin, and I was up and around within the hour. The idea that the discovery of penicillin could have such a powerful impact on health care left a lasting impression on me.

After high school, I spent three pleasant years in the U.S. Army working at Fort Huachuca with scientists and engineers on experimental computers. Then I enrolled at the University of Minnesota with the intent of making a career of medical research. After talking to the medical researchers on campus, I decided to concentrate on a relatively new field: human aging. This was the 1960's, when medical researchers believed they would find a cure for cancer and heart disease in the next 10 years. I concluded that by concentrating on human aging, I would always have a job.

Experiments on Aging Reversal

After graduating from the University of Minnesota with a degree in chemistry and math, I began working at the Sansum Foundation, a gerontological aging research laboratory in Santa Barbara. It was here the work, that led to the human copper-peptide complex GHK-Cu, first emerged during my attempts to reverse detrimental changes that occur during human aging. My goal was to suppress the synthesis of the blood fibrinogen, a blood protein that rises with age and that is an excellent predictor of mortality. Elevated fibrinogen levels increase blood coagulation and decrease tissue nutrition by increasing the thickness of blood in the capillaries.

To understand these changes, I compared the synthesis of fibrinogen in liver biopsy samples from young patients in their 20's with those of patients from 60 to 80 years of age. As expected, the liver tissue from the older group produced more fibrinogen. However, if tissue from the older patients was incubated in the blood from the younger group, it functioned in nearly the same way as the younger liver tissue. Conversely, incubation of the younger liver tissue with blood from the older patients changed the synthesis pattern to that of older tissue. The natural conclusion was that a factor in young blood caused the older tissue to act like younger tissue. GHK-Cu in human blood declines about 60% between age 20 and age 60. This may be a reason for the decrease in tissue repair and viability as we get older.[1]

I isolated this factor while completing my PhD. thesis in biochemistry[2] in M. Michael Thaler's lab at the University of California at San Francisco. The factor turned out to contain a small peptide called glycyl-histidyl-lysine, or GHK, plus another unknown factor. The chemical structure of GHK looked like a copper-binding site, and an analysis by Merle Millard of the Department of Agriculture Labs (Albany, California) found copper in the extracts, so we knew that the active material was a copper-peptide complex. (It was later discovered that GHK obtains its copper from the albumin protein).[3]

In 1974, Boris Weinstein of the University of Washington Chemistry Department wrote to me to suggest that he, an organic chemist, and colleague Norman Rose, an inorganic chemist, could collaborate to determine what role GHK-Cu played in the human body. I decided to focus my efforts on GHK-Cu's actions on cells and tissues[4] while the Seattle group established the chemical properties of the molecule.[5]

Proof of GHK's structure was established by David Schlesinger[6] of the Harvard University Chemistry Department, while Helen Sage[7] of Providence Hospital in Seattle established that GHK is generated by protein breakdown after injury. Groups at the University of Washington, Toronto Hospital for Sick Children[8], and the Albert Einstein Medical School[9] defined the detailed interactions of GHK with the copper 2+ ion. In the body, both GHK and GHK-Cu co-exist, so both structures may have biological actions.[10]

In 1980, I moved to Seattle to continue my work at the Virginia Mason Research Center. By 1983, I had discovered that GHK-Cu accelerates wound healing and contraction, improves the take of transplanted skin[11], and also possesses anti-inflammatory actions. Numerous other laboratories later confirmed the wound-healing actions of GHK-Cu.[12]

Remodeling and a Cat Named Collagen

In 1985, Barbara Weinstein and I started a company called Procyte to develop these findings into useful products. Mrs. Weinstein was the widow of my colleague Boris Weinstein, who was one of the most decent and cultured men I have ever met, and who tragically passed away too early.

Friends are needed to start a small company. John Majnarich, a biochemist whose laboratory researched and produced fish vaccines for salmon farms, offered me free space to start Procyte and again later for Skin Biology.

Between 1986 and 1990, I found that creams containing GHK-Cu, when applied to human skin, increased the thickness of the dermis and epidermis, increased skin elasticity, reduced wrinkles, and resulted in the removal of skin imperfections, such as blotchiness and sun damage marks, while producing an increase in subcutaneous fat cells. But these were small studies and were not pursued at that time.[13]

Around the same time, H. Paul Ehrlich of Shriner's Burn Center in Boston noted with puzzlement that GHK-Cu simultaneously increased both collagen synthesis and collagen breakdown during the healing of wounds.[14]

The major breakthrough on SRCPs and skin remodeling came from the biochemistry group at the University of Reims in France[15]. In 1985, my wife and I were attending a scientific conference in Rome when we met Jacque-Paul Borel and his wife Nadine. My observations on GHK-Cu and wound healing sparked Borel's interest, whose research focused on collagen metabolism to the point that his family's cat was named Collagen. Over the next 14 years, his research group (later headed by Francois Maquart) unraveled many key actions of GHK-Cu on cells critical to skin repair. They observed that, as GHK-Cu triggers the synthesis of messenger RNAs (mRNAs) for metalloproteinases that dissolve scar tissue and damaged skin proteins, it simultaneously induces the production of mRNAs for skin proteins and water-holding molecules (collagen, elastin, proteoglycans, glycosaminoglycans, etc.) needed to rebuild the skin's extracellular matrix after injury. Ultimately, they concluded that GHK-Cu functions to activate the skin's remodeling processes.[15]

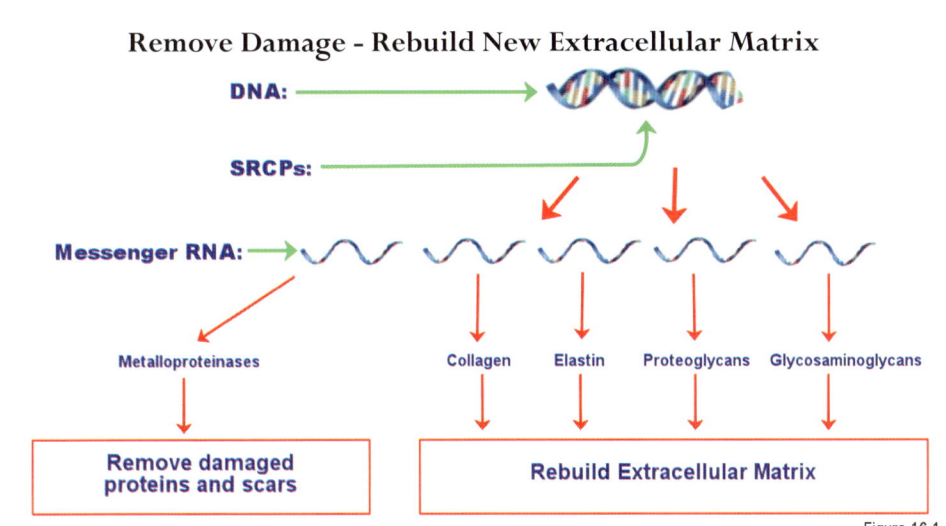

Remove Damage - Rebuild New Extracellular Matrix

Figure 16.1

Also at the University of Reims, Bernard Kalis (dermatology) and Marc Leutenegger (diabetology) treated 60 patients and found that GHK-Cu creams gave strong evidence of the accelerated healing of skin ulcers. Unfortunately, this type of apparently successful healing cream was never tested in larger FDA clinical trials on indolent skin ulcers.[16]

Skin Remodeling: Messages from the Molecule

Skin remodeling was once thought of simply as the process by which scar tissue associated with the early stages of healing was removed and replaced with normal skin. But experiments on GHK-Cu have indicated that remodeling is in fact a far more complex and coordinated process. Most surprising is the indication that GHK-Cu possesses a diverse multiplicity of actions connected with skin remodeling. These actions are described as follows.

Anti-inflammatory Action

In 1984, I observed that GHK-Cu possesses a mild antioxidant activity similar to the enzyme superoxide dismutase, which manifests itself as a calming of red and irritated skin. Steve Aust's lab at Utah State University subsequently discovered that GHK-Cu blocks the damage-induced release of oxidizing iron molecules from ferritin. Aust also said SRCPs did a great job of healing wounds in his horses.

Further discoveries followed. Vicini and colleagues at the University of Catalina in Italy reported that GHK-Cu blocks tissue damage by Interleukin-1. Then, Robert Koch's lab at Stanford University reported that GHK-Cu shuts down the production, by normal and keloid fibroblasts, of the scar-forming protein TGF-ß-1. Interestingly, they also found that retinoic acid, which is thought to trigger remodeling, actually increases this scar-forming factor.[17]

Re-establishment of Blood Flow

GHK-Cu helps re-establish blood flow into damaged tissues through a mixture of three actions: angiogenesis, anti-coagulation, and vasodilation. GHK-Cu increases the expression of basic fibroblast growth factor and vascular endothelial growth factor, both of which aid blood vessel formation.[18] GHK-Cu-induced angiogenesis (new blood-vessel formation) was documented by Pietro Guillo's lab at the National Cancer Institute in Bethesda.[19]

At Providence Heart Center in Seattle, Lester Savage's lab found that GHK-Cu inhibited platelet aggregation and the formation of vasoconstrictive thromboxane, an action that may reduce localized blood coagulation after tissue damage. My lab, in turn, discovered that the intravenous perfusion of GHK-Cu into goats produces a dramatic fall in blood pressure, while Leslie Manot of the University of Reims found that GHK-Cu's vasodilation actions increases blood flow in perfused hearts.[20]

The vasodilation action may arise from GHK's binding to the angiotensin II receptor in the same way as many vasodilatory drugs, such as Losartan.

GHK-Cu may also increase the production of erythropoietin which stimulates red blood cell production.[21]

Chemoattraction, Repair, and Skin Contraction

GHK-Cu is a powerful attractant for capillary cells that build new blood vessels, an action that was discovered by my lab. At Harvard University, Bruce Zetter's lab found similar actions of GHK-Cu on macrophages and mast cells. Macrophages remove damaged cellular debris and secrete a cornucopia of 20 or more proteins (fibroblasts growth factor, epidermal growth factor, and so on) important for healing in the area of tissue damage.[22] Mast cells stimulate skin contraction. In earlier wound-healing experiments, I observed GHK-Cu to both heal wounds and induce a powerful skin contraction around the wound.

Promotion of Nerve Outgrowth

When wound healing is inadequate, the healed area is often devoid of sensory abilities. In cell cultures, both Monique Sensenbrenner's lab at the University of Strasbourg in France and Gertrude Lindler's lab at Karl Marx University in Berlin, Germany found that GHK stimulates nerve outgrowth, an essential attribute of skin repair. Ahmed and colleagues at the Neurochemistry Lab in Chennai, India wrote that when severed nerves are placed in a collagen tube impregnated with GHK, there is an increased production of nerve growth factor and the neurotrophins NT-3 and NT-4.[23]

Hair Follicles and Stem Cells

During World War II, physicians discovered that after burns to the skin, when hair follicles appeared at the edge of the healing wound, scar-free healing followed. If no follicles were observed, healing was incomplete and the scar remained. Likewise, when I studied the morphology of experimental wounds treated with GHK-Cu, the wound edge always was filled with enlarged hair follicles with greatly enlarged sebaceous glands. Yet there was no logical connection between hair follicles and skin repair. Then in 2000, a research group in Paris broadened our understanding of healing skin when they reported that stem cells for skin are secreted from enlarged sebaceous glands protruding from the enlarged hair follicles.[24]

HAIR FOLLICLES and STEM CELLS
Human Hair: 98% Vellus Hairs
2% Terminal Hairs

Vellus Hair Follicles

Produces nearly invisible, fine, short hairs on the skin
(4.8 - 4.9 million on body)

SRCPs increase follicle size ➡

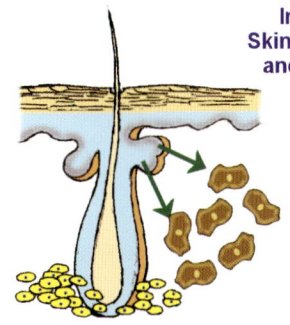

RESULT:
Improved Skin Rebuilding and Renewal

Produces Stem Cells for Skin

Terminal Hair Follicles

Produces long, thick, visible hairs on the skin
(100,000 - 150,000 on body)

SRCPs increase follicle size ➡

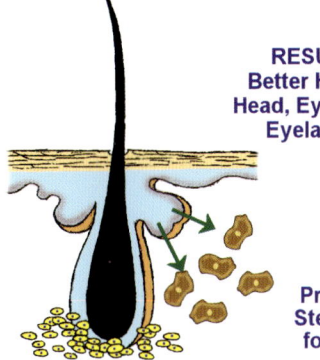

RESULT:
Better Hair on Head, Eyebrows, Eyelashes

Produces Stem Cells for Scalp

SRCPs increase follicle size, but vellus follicles are **not** changed into terminal (long-hair) follicles. The use of SRCP facial products does **not** result in increased facial hair.

Figure 16.2

Remodeling of Aged Skin

My early observations that GHK-Cu could reverse the skin damage that accumulates during aging gathered dust for a decade. Finally, between 1998 and 2002, more extensive human studies solidified my observations. Abulghani et al. reported that GHK-Cu was more effective in stimulating new collagen development than vitamin C, retinoic acid, or melatonin. Appa et al. reported, following an eight-week study, that a GHK-containing liquid foundation improved epidermal thickness, increased skin elasticity, and improved skin appearance. Leydan et al. found, in another eight week study, that such creams reduced the visible signs of photo damage and increased skin density on facial skin. In a further, placebo-controlled study involving 71 females over 12 weeks, GHK-Cu was found to reduce wrinkles and fine lines while increasing the skin's elasticity, density, and thickness. Another placebo-controlled study, involving 41 females over 12 weeks, found that GHK-Cu in eye cream reduced wrinkles and fine lines and improved eye appearance. GHK-Cu also strongly increased keratinocyte proliferation in women over age 50 with photo-damaged skin, improved overall appearance, and tightened loose skin.[25]

Mechanism of Skin Repair and Remodeling

After decades of research, here's how I propose skin repair and remodeling works based on our current knowledge.

1. After skin damage, the body's damage control mechanisms stop blood loss (if any), then cover the damaged skin with a layer of tough protective scar tissue. A type of immune cell, the neutrophil, quickly arrives in the damaged area and sterilizes it by releasing toxic oxygen radicals to kill bacteria. This action is usually very brief, but occasionally the damage continues and the skin becomes chronically inflamed. The tissue-damaging cytokine Interleukin-1 may cause further damage.

2. The protein TGF-ß-1 is produced to stimulate scar production. Large amounts of scar-forming collagen are secreted into the damaged area.

3. The skin damage also causes the release of enzymes that break down damaged skin proteins into smaller peptide fragments. Copper ions accumulate in the wound area and combine with special peptides to form SRCPs. If the skin is copper deficient, healing will be inadequate. The copper peptides serve as chemical signals to the immune system that the skin is injured and needs repair.

4. The SRCPs then initiate the skin remodeling. Scar tissue is removed and replaced with normal tissue. As the SRCPs accumulate, they act directly to protect the tissues by (a) blocking the release of tissue-damaging iron from ferritin, (b) increasing the level of protective superoxide dismutase activities, and (c) suppressing the scar formation by inhibiting the production of TGF-ß-1 and blocking the actions of Interleukin-1.

5. SRCPs also attract other immune cells. Macrophages arrive and remove the skin debris produced by the damage and secrete about 20 different growth factors needed for proper skin repair. These have names such as epidermal growth factor, fibroblast growth factor, platelet-derived growth factor, and so on. The macrophage action helps remove chronically damaged, abnormal skin, such as spots and lesions from sun damage. Mast cells also arrive and speed skin tightening.

6. SRCPs then stimulate the production of the body's scar-removal systems by activating the synthesis of metalloproteinases (a family of at least 14 proteins that remove damaged proteins, such as damaged collagen and elastin) and antiproteases. At the same time, SRCPs activate the creation of new collagen and elastin to give the skin strength and elasticity, and other proteins such as proteoglycans and glycosaminoglycans that bind large amounts of water to moisturize the skin.

7. SRCPs re-establish blood angiogenesis (new capillary formation) and vasodilate new blood vessels to nourish and oxygenate the newly repaired skin while inhibiting blood coagulation.

8. SRCPs also promote nerve outgrowth into the repaired area.

9. SRCPs increase the size of the skins vellus hair follicles. New stem cells arise from the hair follicle and migrate into the surrounding skin area. A great proliferation of fibroblasts and keratinocytes follows as scar tissue is removed and the skin is restored to its pre-damage condition.

10. SRCPs may increase the production of erythropoietin, which increases red blood cells.

11. Skin remodeling continues for a long period to slowly restore the skin to its original condition.

Proposed Actions of GHK-Cu on Skin
(Based on Published Articles)

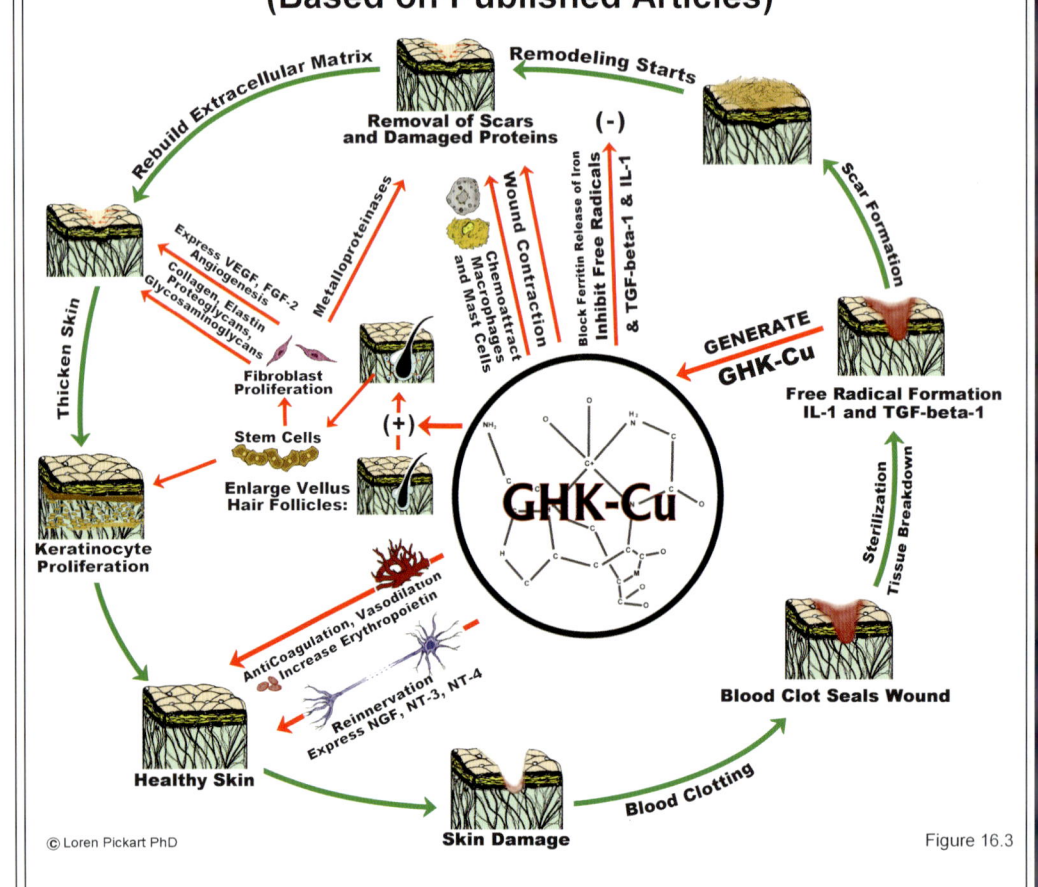

Figure 16.3

© Loren Pickart PhD

Second-Generation SRCPs

Although the first-generation of products containing GHK-Cu performed well in many tests, they failed FDA clinical trials on difficult-to-heal human wounds, such as skin ulcers (as have many other approaches). GHK-Cu's actions are limited by fragility and a tendency toward breakdown, as well as a lack of adhesion to the skin's surface.

As I was working on these problems, a blood clot in an airport and a slow recovery from heart surgery forced me to leave Procyte. But this gave me more time to think about better approaches to copper-based tissue repair.

To find a better method, first I bought a boat and named it Regenerate, then spent time studying skin repair while cruising and fishing around the islands of Washington State and British Columbia.

Figure 16.4

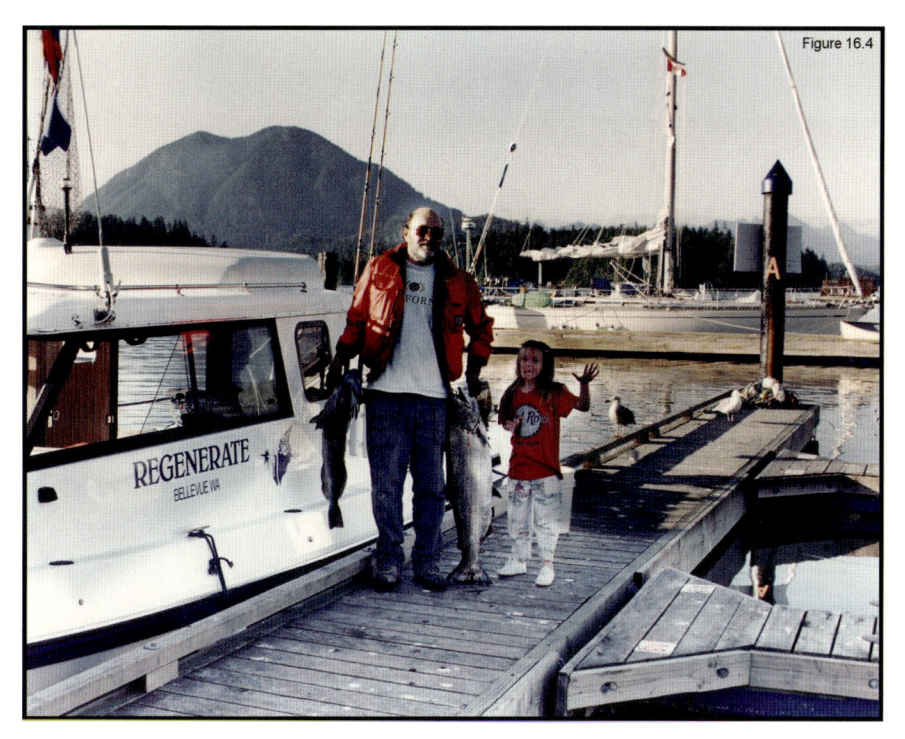

I theorized that after skin damage, the body's breakdown processes generate a blizzard of small peptides, including GHK, in the damaged area. Since GHK has a very strong affinity to bind copper (II) ions and can obtain copper ion from tissue fluids, it occurred to me that other small peptides might act as SRCPs if pre-loaded with copper ions. Therefore, in 1994 my wife Charlene and I started Skin Biology to develop improved second-generation skin regenerative/remodeling copper peptides with enhanced potency, breakdown resistance, and high adherence to skin.

To accomplish this goal, I isolated peptide fragments from soy protein digests that possessed the desired qualities when chelated to copper (II). Such peptides have a long history of safe use in cosmetic products. In human and veterinary studies, creams made from these new copper complexes showed superior healing actions in all of my standard tests. They accelerated wound closure, produced greatly enlarged hair follicles, possessed anti-inflammatory actions as good as cortisone, increased the synthesis of collagen and elastin, and produced rapid and scar-free healing in dogs after spaying operations and in young horses after leg straightening operations.[26]

Howard Maibach of the University of California San Francisco and colleagues also tested the second-generation copper peptides in four small placebo-controlled human studies. They found that creams made from the new copper complexes produced significantly faster skin healing and reduced redness and inflammation after mild skin injuries brought on by tape stripping, acetone burns (removal of skin lipids), 24-hour detergent irritation, and nickel allergy inflammation.[27]

While the second-generation SRCPs were originally developed to help prevent skin damage in nursing homes and hospitals, somewhat accidentally, women and men began using them on their skin and reporting back good results. Excitingly, the breakdown-resistant SRCPs can be used with hydroxy acids and retinoic acid to enhance skin remodeling and the removal of many types of blemishes and scars.

Other Uses of SRCPs

While the proceeding discussion focused on skin actions, research has determined that SRCPs have many other positive effects on the hair and other parts of the body, as follows.

Repair Signal for Many Organs

GHK-Cu has been found to trigger repair in many types of tissues, such as the hair system, stomach lining, gastrointestinal tract, bones, and liver.

Improved Hair Growth and Condition

In 1985 I observed that, after treating skin wounds with GHK-Cu, there was a profound enlargement of the hair follicles at the wound edge. Further work with radioisotopes indicated that SRCPs were present at the site of injection for only about 30 seconds before being cleared from the area. This meant that a very brief exposure of the hair follicle to SRCPs was sufficient to produce an increase in follicle volume. Such an exposure increased hair growth in mice four- to eight-fold within 12 days, as the following photos demonstrate.

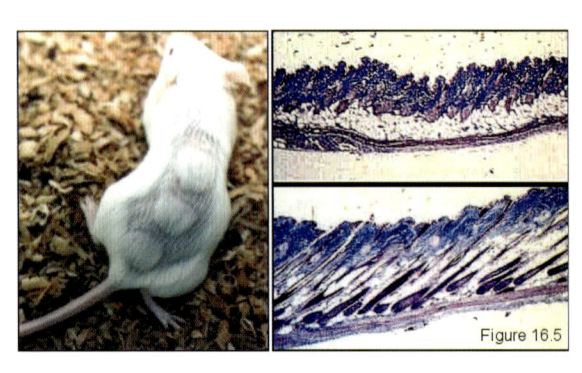

NORMAL HAIR FOLLICLES

ENLARGED HAIR FOLLICLES:
(After injection of SRCPs)

Figure 16.5

A 25 day-old mouse was shaved and injected intradermally in three spots with a SRCP. Twelve days later, there was a very strong stimulation of hair growth at the injection sites.

Further work by myself and Steven Lovejoy of the University of Washington found that the chemical addition of fat-like molecules, such as fatty acids or hydrophobic amino acid residues, to GHK-Cu resulted in an intensified follicle enlargement action and stimulation of hair growth in undamaged mouse skin. [28]

These discoveries were extended by Hideo Uno at the University of Wisconsin. Uno had written The UpJohn Company's textbook for physicians when Rogaine® (minoxidil) first was marketed. [29]

Bernard Kalis of the University of Reims was the first researcher to demonstrate that SRCPs have positive actions in humans. His studies found SRCPs caused a greater proportion of human follicles to switch from the dormant telogen state into the hair-growing anagen state. [30] A later, placebo-controlled, three-month study in male humans found that a SRCP (Ala-His-Lys: copper(II)) in a product called Tricomin® increased the number of terminal hairs and was 32 percent more effective than a control group that used 2 percent minoxidil. [31]

Improved Hair Transplantation

In addition to stimulating hair growth, SRCPs have been shown to improve human hair transplantation. When used in the post-operative regimen, GraftCyte®, a SRCP product sold by ProCyte, results in faster healing of transplants and earlier regrowth of the hair shafts. Studies by Perez-Meza and colleagues found that the GraftCyte system provided enhanced healing of the transplanted follicles and more immediate hair growth. In their study, patients saw new hair growth in six weeks, versus the normal 10 to 14 weeks. In most cases, skin crusting after transplantation is reduced from 10 to 14 days to five days.

A second study of GraftCyte by Gary Hitzig, involving 30 hair transplant patients, found that GraftCyte reduced the shedding of transplanted hair from 30 percent with saline to 10 percent with Graftcyte. The healing time of the transplanted grafts was cut in half. Regrowth of new hair from the transplants occurred in six to eight weeks with saline and four to six weeks with Graftcyte. Patient satisfaction after transplantation rose from 80 percent to 95 percent. [32] GraftCyte can be ordered from www.procyte.com.

Accelerated Hair Regrowth after Chemotherapy

Studies by Awa and Nogimori of Kaken Pharmaceuticals in Japan reported that pre-treatment of mice with SRCPs blocked the hair loss induced by the cancer chemotherapy drugs cytosine arabinoside and doxorubicin. If the mice were first treated with chemotherapeutic drugs to induce hair loss, subsequent treatment with SRCPs accelerated the recovery of lost hair. [33]

At Skin Biology, the second-generation SRCPs also strongly stimulated hair growth in mice. To enhance the uptake of SRCPs into the hair follicles, natural penetrating agents, such as emu oil and squalane from olives, were used to push more SRCPs into the follicle area.

Restoration of Damaged Liver

Researchers at Kursk Medical University in Russia found that in rats, GHK increased the replication of hepatocytes while decreasing hepatic immune reactivity (delayed hypersensitivity reaction). After acute toxic damage to the liver caused by tetrachloromethane, intraperitoneal administration of GHK restored normal liver functions and immune responsiveness.[34]

Reduction of Stomach Ulcers and Intestinal Damage

In rat ulcer models, GHK-Cu, given orally, reduced gastric acidity, increased mucous production, and inhibited the development of gastric ulcers. Likewise, in intestinal duodenal ulcer models, GHK-Cu inhibited ulcer development.[35] One study of 16 human patients with distal inflammatory bowel disease, who were treated with rectally administered solutions of GHK-Cu, found that after the 12 weeks of treatment, there was a 60 percent reduction in severity as measured by endoscopy, histopathology, and symptoms.[36]

Accelerated Bone Healing

GHK-Cu accelerates the healing of bones by increasing the formation of healing granulation tissue in damaged bones. GHK-Cu has also been shown to increase collagen synthesis by bone chondrocytes from chickens and pigs, increase the growth of human marrow stromal cells, and promote the attachment of human osteoblastic cells.

Milan Adam's group at the Medical University in Prague developed a GHK-Cu gel that was shown to promote the filling of bone defects in femurs and bone attachment to cementless endoprostheses. The GHK-Cu gel, when used with cementless endoprotheses, produced vivid osteogenic activity at the interface of bone and metal stem. Such gels may aid in the establishment and retention of artificial joints.[37]

The Future of GHK-Cu

GHK-Cu remains the best molecule for internal medical treatments. The newer breakdown-resistant, highly adhesive copper peptides under development at Skin Biology should prove better for cosmetic and superficial uses, such as postprocedure dermatological healing and development of scarless surgical procedures.

It is possible that in the future, GHK-Cu will be used clinically to protect and speed the repair of damaged organs. H. Paul Ehrlich found that intra-muscular injection of GHK-Cu into the thigh muscle in rabbits raised circulating wound macrophages in the blood and accelerated the healing of distant wounds in the rabbits ear.[14,38] Someday, patients may be pre-treated with GHK-Cu before surgery to enhance post-surgery repair. Based on rabbit models, a very safe dosage of 30 mg of GHK-Cu should suffice. This is about 700-fold below the level of potential toxic actions of GHK-Cu. (A sudden increase in blood GHK-Cu levels produces a drastic fall in blood pressure presumably due to vasodilation actions).

It appears GHK-Cu can be used for the biological repair of a variety of tissues. We know that the molecule helps damaged skin, dysfunctional hair follicles, the gastrointestinal tract, the liver, and the bones, but it may have repair properties on many other tissues and organs as well. For example, GHK-Cu is very beneficial on kidney and lung organ cultures.[39] One day, GHK-Cu might be infused into patients with kidney failure to exert its tissue protective and repair actions. Other areas of interest include damaged nerve tissue, inflamed lungs, and knee and hip joints. Some people with gum problems tell me they brush their teeth with SRCPs and have good results.

The current trend in medicine is to replace defective body parts with plastic and metal devices. Biological tissue repair, using the body's natural mechanisms, would be far superior.

TISSUE REPAIR BY GHK-Cu

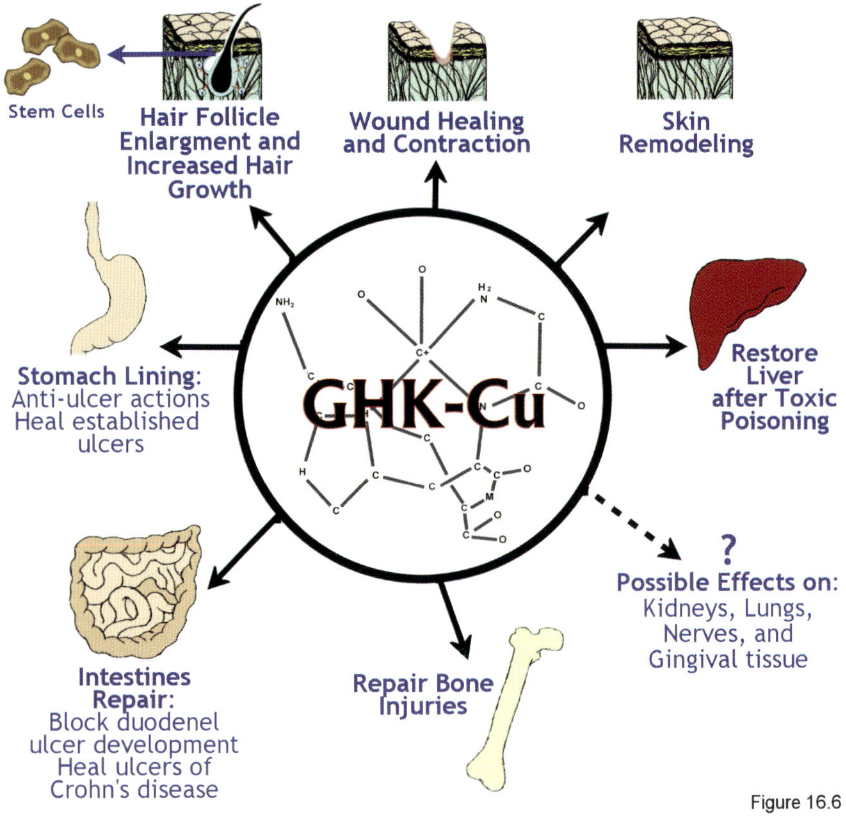

Stem Cells

Hair Follicle Enlargment and Increased Hair Growth

Wound Healing and Contraction

Skin Remodeling

Stomach Lining: Anti-ulcer actions Heal established ulcers

GHK-Cu

Restore Liver after Toxic Poisoning

Intestines Repair: Block duodenel ulcer development Heal ulcers of Crohn's disease

Repair Bone Injuries

? Possible Effects on: Kidneys, Lungs, Nerves, and Gingival tissue

Figure 16.6

Chapter 17

COPPER:

Your Body's Protective & Anti-Aging Metal

Some 2,000 years ago, the ancients referred to copper as the metal of healing and the metal of love. They were right on both counts. Since SRCPs contain copper, our clients often ask about the safety and function of copper within the body.

Copper is an essential metal necessary for many body processes. Copper deficiency is thought to contribute to a host of health problems, including a higher rate of: cellular oxidation, cancer, cardiovascular disease, atherosclerosis, LDL "bad cholesterol", lipid oxidation, aortic aneurysms, osteoarthritis, rheumatoid arthritis, osteoporosis, chronic conditions involving bone and connective tissue, brain defects in newborns, obesity, graying of hair, sensitivity to pain, Alzheimer's disease, reproductive problems, depression, and fatigue; as well as lower HDL "good cholesterol", reduction in the pleasure producing brain enkephalins, and impaired brain function.

The Two Forms of Copper

In the human body, copper moves between the cuprous (copper (I) or Cu 1+) form and the cupric (copper (II) or Cu 2+) form. Copper (II) is the form of copper that induces tissue regeneration and skin repair. It gives a blue color in water and a blue-to-green color when formulated into creams, lotions, and solutions. Copper (I) has no tissue regenerative or skin-repair activity and is colorless in water.

Most of the body's copper is bound into proteins where it plays an important role in biological activities, such as antioxidant effects, energy generation, and tissue regeneration. A very small fraction, less that 1 percent, known as metabolically active copper, is exchanged between the various tissues of the body as needed and is bound either to amino acids, peptides, or proteins. This exchangeable copper is an indicator of good health: its level is high in healthy people, but diminishes in those with inflammatory diseases, such as arthritis.

How Much Copper Do You Need?

Most nutritionists recommend a daily copper dosage that ranges from 1 to 3 mg, but there is no certainty to this number. Many scientists who study copper and health take 4 mg daily of supplemental copper. Studies in humans have found that daily supplemental copper, ranging from 4 to 7 mg, has positive actions, such as reducing damaging cellular oxidation, lowering LDL levels, and increasing HDL levels. Such higher intakes may reduce the risk of some degenerative diseases, but nutritionists also recommend not exceeding 10 mg of copper daily.

Copper deficiency diseases are virtually the same as the pattern of major degenerative diseases in the U.S. The one condition where copper intake must be restricted is Wilson's disease, a rare genetic condition that affects 1,600 people in the U.S.

Something to consider is that since copper and zinc compete for uptake in the body, a high copper intake reduces zinc absorption, and, conversely, a high zinc intake reduces copper absorption. Thus, a balance should be maintained between these two metals. The best guess is that the ratio of seven parts by weight of zinc to one part copper is adequate. In addition to taking a copper supplement, another way to boost your daily intake of copper is by eating copper-rich foods. These include seafood, shellfish, liver, nuts, seeds, beans, whole-grain breads, cocoa, and chocolate.

Uptake of Copper from SRCP Products

Very little copper from SRCP products, only about 0.1 percent or less, penetrates the skin. Charged molecules, including copper and peptides, have very poor penetration of the skin. Numerous safety studies of SRCP products have failed to find a rise in blood copper or any other negative action.

So don't worry about factoring the copper from copper-peptide products into your daily copper intake. If you were to use two grams of copper-peptide product daily that contained 2 mg of copper, assuming the skin uptake was at 0.1 percent penetration, this would introduce only about 0.002 mg of copper into your body.

More Support for a Copper-Rich Diet

The copper-containing protein copper-zinc superoxide dismutase (CuZnSOD) is the primary antioxidant defense in the human body. Higher levels of CuZnSOD are a major factor in a longer lifespan in animals. However, because copper (II) is usually in short supply in the human body, CuZnSOD has only about 50 percent of the copper it needs (zinc supplies are usually adequate). This shortage markedly reduces CuZnSOD's antioxidant powers and is another reason why a higher level of dietary copper is beneficial.

While CuZnSOD requires two metals, copper and zinc, only copper seems to regulate the antioxidant activity. Restricting dietary copper quickly impairs the catalytic function of CuZnSOD in numerous tissues. However, when diets are supplemented with copper, the CuZnSOD activity is quickly restored.[1]

Animal studies have found that a reduced copper intake increases deleterious cellular oxidation and promotes a wide variety of the types of degenerative diseases associated with aging. On the other hand, a higher dietary copper intake in animals reduces overall damaging cellular oxidation.

The good health of people who live in certain high mountain valleys around the world offers additional support for a higher dietary copper intake. People living in the Hunza area of Pakistan, the Vilcabamba area of Ecuador, the Caucasus area of Georgia, Northwest Tibet, and the Titicaca area of the Peruvian Andes all have very different diets but drink the same hard water from glaciers, which has a very high mineral content. In all of these regions, the lifespan and health of the elderly is exceptional. In contrast, regions with soft water that is low in minerals have high rates of cancer and heart disease. In the past, physicians would send their patients to sanatoriums where they drank mineral water and bathed in it.

Confusion Over Copper and Disease

Of the copper in blood serum, only a small fraction is metabolically active. Ninety-five percent is found in the antioxidant protein ceruloplasmin. During many diseases and stress conditions, the body increases ceruloplasmin levels as a protective antioxidant mechanism. Because metabolically active copper is technically difficult to measure, most studies of copper and disease report only the level of copper in the blood serum. This often leads to false conclusions as to the role of copper in disease states.[2]

For example, total blood plasma copper is elevated in diseases such as cancer, heart disease, and arthritis, but this increase is due to increased ceruloplasmin in the blood. Some misinformed individuals have interpreted this increase in blood copper as an indication that a high level of copper causes disease. But when copper supplements are given to animals and humans, the additional dietary copper has been found to lower carcinogenesis and tumor growth, inhibit the development of cardiovascular problems, and reverse many arthritic effects. Most of the rest of this chapter will discuss the impact of copper on various health conditions.

Copper and Cancer

The Center for Disease Control states that Copper has not been shown to cause cancer in people or animals. In fact, there is mounting evidence that copper actually helps fight cancer.

Consider the following. Colon cancer is the second most deadly form of cancer in the U.S. APC, a gene known to suppress the formation of tumors, is mutated during colon cancer development. Individuals possessing these mutations develop numerous intestinal polyps (precancerous lesions). A species of mice have a mutation similar to APC that causes intestinal polyps and colon cancer. Nutritionist Cindy D. Davis of the Human Nutrition Research Center in North Dakota found that when these mice were fed a copper-deficient diet (20 percent lower than normal), they developed a significantly higher small intestine tumor incidence and mass than mice fed adequate dietary copper. Davis says these results have important implications because 80 percent of the population in the United States does not ingest adequate amounts of copper.[3]

Copper complexes cause some types of cancer cells to revert to non-cancerous growth patterns. John R. J. Sorenson of University of Arkansas for Medical Sciences and colleagues treated rats which had solid tumors with various copper complexes (such as copper salicylate) and found that this treatment decreased tumor growth and increased survival rates. These copper complexes did not kill cancer cells, but often caused them to revert to the growth patterns of normal (differentiated) cells.

In another study, Sorenson found that numerous copper complexes with superoxide dismutase activity retarded the spontaneous development of cancers in mice.[4] Copper stimulates the production of the tumor-suppressor protein p53, which inhibits the growth of tumors in the body.[5]

Copper and Cardiovascular Disease

Human and animal studies demonstrate that copper deficiency increases plasma cholesterol, "bad" LDL cholesterol, and blood pressure while decreasing "good" HDL cholesterol, thus increasing the risk of cardiovascular disease.[6]

Investigators have found that copper complexes can minimize damage to the aorta and heart muscle following myocardial infarction. Severe copper deficiency results in heart abnormalities and damage (cardiomyopathy) in some animals.[7]

A multi-center study found that copper supplementation of 3 to 6 mg daily increased the resistance of red blood cells to damaging oxidation, indicating that relatively high intakes of copper do not increase the susceptibility of LDL or red blood cells to oxidation.[8] Rats on a copper-deficient diet had a decrease in aortic integrity that produced eventual aneurysm.[9]

Copper and Immune System Function

A medical publication in 1867 reported that, during the Paris cholera epidemics of 1832, 1849, and 1852, workers exposed to copper salts did not develop cholera. Immune impairment can be detected by one week after the start of a diet low in copper; conversely, the addition of adequate copper rapidly reverses the immune suppression within one week. [10]

Animals deficient in copper have an increased susceptibility to bacterial pathogens such as salmonella and listeria.[10] A study of 11 infants with copper deficiencies found that the ability of their white blood cells to engulf pathogens increased after one month of copper supplementation.[11] Adult men on a low-copper diet (0.66 mg of copper a day for 24 days, and then 0.38 mg a day for another 40 days) showed a decreased ability of mononuclear cells to respond to antigens.[12] Abnormally low numbers of white blood cells is a clinical indicator of copper deficiency in humans and functioning of macrophages decreases in even marginally copper-deficient rats.[13]

Copper and Arthritis

John R. J. Sorenson has led the scientific work on the use of copper complexes to treat patients with arthritic and other chronic degenerative diseases. He has found the copper complexes of more than 140 anti-inflammatory agents, such as aspirin and ibuprofen, to be far more active than these compounds without copper. Copper aspirinate has been shown to be more effective in the treatment of rheumatoid arthritis than aspirin alone. It also has been shown to prevent or even cure the ulceration of the stomach often associated with aspirin therapy.

1885, the French physician Luton effectively treated arthritic patients with a salve of hogs lard and 30 percent neutral copper acetate applied to the skin over affected joints. He also had his patients take pills containing 10 mg of copper acetate.

Studies of rheumatoid arthritis exemplify the paradox that has so confounded researchers on copper and its effects on various diseases. For example, between 1940 and 1970, studies of patients with rheumatoid arthritis found them to have higher than normal serum copper levels. Similar results were found in other various inflammatory diseases in humans and animals. Yet, in seeming contradiction, copper complexes were successfully used in the treatment of numerous conditions characterized by arthritic changes and inflammation.

Subsequent research concluded that an increase in serum copper is a physiological response to inflammation, rather than a cause of inflammation. The rise in copper is due to an elevation of the ceruloplasmin in serum, a protein with strong anti-inflammatory activity. Copper deficiency increases the severity of experimentally induced inflammation.[14]

Copper and Osteoporosis

Two hundred years ago, the German physician Rademacher established that copper supplements speed the healing of broken bones in patients. Inadequate dietary copper causes osteoporosis in numerous animal species and humans. Copper deficiency is also associated with scoliosis, skeletal abnormalities, and increased susceptibility to fractures. Inadequate dietary copper lowers bone calcium levels.

A study of elderly subjects found a decreased loss of bone-mineral density from the lumbar spine after copper supplementation of 3 mg daily for two years. Healthy adult males on a low-copper intake (0.7 mgs daily) for six weeks exhibited an increased rate of bone breakdown.[15]

Anti-convulsant Activities of Copper Complexes

The brain contains more copper than any other organ except the liver, where copper is stored for use elsewhere. This fact suggests that copper plays a role in brain functions. Due to seizures in animals and humans during the consumption of copper-deficient diets, it was subsequently discovered many anti-convulsant drugs are more effective and less toxic when complexed with copper.[16]

Copper and Pregnancy

In the 1930's, at a sheep station in Western Australia, many newborn lambs were uncoordinated, had difficulty standing, and subsequently died. Later it was determined that the pregnant sheep were pastured on land that produced grass with a very low copper content. The grass didn't provide enough copper for normal development of the lamb's nervous systems and brains.

Research at the US Department of Agriculture's Grand Forks Human Nutrition Research Center found that even marginal copper deficiency in pregnant rats produces brain damage and neurological defects in their offspring. The newborn rats have structural abnormalities in the areas of the brain involved in learning and memory and those responsible for coordination and movement. These abnormalities resulted in behavioral changes, for example, the young rats lacked the normal startle reflex to unexpected noises. The copper deficit permanently affected the young rats and could not be corrected by a high-copper diet.

Another study reported that copper deficiency during pregnancy can result in numerous gross structural and biochemical abnormalities, which seem to arise because the copper deficiency reduces free radical defense mechanisms, connective tissue metabolism, and energy production.[17]

Copper and Protein Glycation

One of the deleterious changes with age is an increased attachment of sugars to protein, known as protein glycation. This process produces less functional proteins. An increased copper intake has been found to reduce protein glycation.[18]

Does the Copper in Wine Help the French Live Longer?

Citizens of France are blessed with exceptionally healthy lives; they are some of the longest-lived people on earth and have a very low rate of heart disease despite their traditionally high-fat diet. Some researchers have speculated that the low heart-attack rate in France compared to the rest of Europe is due to the heavy drinking of red wine by the French. It is worth noting that there is copper in red wine from the skin of the grapes, which retain copper from the sulfates used by French vintners. Red wine from France contains about 0.2 mg of copper per liter.

Copper and Love

The proceeding establishes the role of copper as the Metal of Healing. But what about the ancient description of copper as the Metal of Love? Sorenson determined that copper complexes reduce pain and may activate opioid receptors. Also, increased tissue copper has been found to increase brain enkephalins and endorphins, our pleasure-creating opiod-like molecules.[19]

The hormone DHEA is converted into the sexual hormones, testosterone and estrogen, and protects the body from the damaging actions of cortisol. DHEA levels sharply decrease with age, while cortisol is relatively constant. This means that tissues are more easily damaged by excess cortisol and we are more stressed while our sexual hormones diminish.

DHEA is widely used as a dietary supplement to help prevent deleterious changes with age. Klevay and Christopherson found that copper deficiency in rats decreased DHEA in serum by approximately 50 percent. The researchers suggest that eating a higher-copper diet increases the DHEA level in the body.[20]

So what about the Metal of Love? While an endorphin-induced sense of euphoric pleasure, coupled with feeling less stress and high personal sexual hormones, may not be love, it is still a good approximation.

Ancient Ideas Rise Again

Modern Spiritualists, like those several thousand years ago, have again focused on copper. As with most of their beliefs, Spiritualists have taken a true scientific property of a mineral and made it to fit their own structure. Because copper is a good physical conductor of electricity and heat, copper is the conductor of the Spiritualist's belief system. According to their myths, copper has the ability to conduct spiritual energy back and forth from individuals, crystals, auras, the mind and the spirit world. They also believe it has the power to amplify thoughts in receiving and sending psychic communication and is used in channeling hoaxes throughout the world. New Age followers also carry it with their stones and crystals to "straighten" the properties of the crystals and use it when creating crystal wands used to connect to spirits, and for channeling spirits and increasing cosmic awareness. It is also instrumental in their physical and mental healing rites.

> *"But couldn't everyone's life become a work of art?
> Why should the lamp or the house be an art object,
> but not your life?"*
> — Michel Foucault

Chapter 18

The Moral Need for Beauty

Do you delight in your quest for beauty or do you feel vain? I once knew a woman who lamented with me in jest. As she applied shiny lacquer to plump her lips, she laughed: "I'm vain. I sit here at my vanity table full of vanity items and primp myself in vain." And indeed her vanity table was adorned with exotic bottles of colorful lotions and cosmetic potions (many of which were useless concoctions as we've discussed earlier). However, I assured her that her quest for beautiful skin and hair was not only natural, it was a moral need she inherited from women throughout the ages. It was in her genes. And like many people, she was a bit embarrassed about the price tag of her costly cosmetics. Maybe this was what Shakespeare meant by "unthrifty loveliness" in Sonnet 4. "I feel shallow," she added. However that didn't stop her from applying a lush coat of mascara. I reassured her that there was nothing shallow about the quest for beauty.

Women decorate their homes and receive praise, but don't want to admit how many hours spent trying to look one's best. The pursuit of beauty is nothing to be ashamed of. After all, glowing skin and shiny hair have always been associated with good health. So in a sense, the quest for beauty is really the quest for health in all its wonderful aspects.

Good health aside, who can deny the pleasure we receive when gazing at men and women who put themselves together well? It's not about looking like a supermodel, but rather about taking the time to enhance your own unique assets, to be the very best you can be. It may take a little time, but aren't you worth it?

Cosmetics, Jewelry, Technology, Art, Symbolism

So OK, maybe your vanity table brims over with a plethora of products. But don't let that turn into unease about your personal vanity. There are those in our society who equate the obsession with self-beauty as some type of moral defect or evil. Deeply caring about the beauty of the human body is an essential part of a tight matrix of behaviors that create what is best in humans. The most valued possessions of early humans were cosmetic body paints such as red ochre (a form of iron ore), jewelry such as necklaces made from small seashells or fox teeth, a technology that created finely crafted tools such as arrowheads, spear points, and implements for food preparation and sewing, and symbolic figurative art objects and geometric forms. The behavior that creates these objects rises from the deepest recesses of the human psyche. We cannot function properly without them. Red lipstick and computer microprocessors arise from the same deep human drives and needs.

The human body, itself, has been a vessel for artistic expression for hundreds of thousands of years. In all civilizations where art, science, and culture have flourished, women and men found ways to embellish their beauty. And like literature, which reveals inner truth through poetic metaphor, outer beauty can reflect the beauty within. It's our moral right and need to look and feel our best.

It's In Your Genes

Mutual grooming, rubbing, and caressing of skin exists in all social animals. Some birds and primates spend up to 90 percent of their time grooming themselves or others. Humans are no different; the drive for beauty is innate to our DNA code. Grooming and working on your skin, nails, and hair increases your body's level of "happiness hormones" or endorphins that increase your sense of well being. Being groomed by someone else increases your endorphins the most.

All early human cultures showed signs of being obsessed with personal beauty. Painting the skin, piercing various body parts, and wearing natural materials including bones, feathers, and shells in the holes was practiced by young and old alike. Ninety-nine percent of our ancestors lived in small nomadic bands of hunters and gatherers, and our psychological drives still reflect this. In ancient times, smooth skin and thick, shiny hair contributed to reproductive success—the reason why these qualities appeal to us today.

Body Painting: The First Make-up

Body painting may be the deepest and most fundamental luxury behavior of humans. Collections of red ochre by humans date back to at least 285,000 years. In Africa, people have been wearing necklaces and using body paints for more than 75,000 years. Skeletons sprinkled with red ochre have been found in graves dating as far back as the Paleolithic Period, when northern Europe was still covered by ice sheets and humans were hunters and gatherers. This ancient burial ritual suggests that body painting was already a long-established practice among the living. Minerals from the earth, chiefly ochre in shades ranging from red to yellow and pyrolosite (manganese) in shades of black and white, were used as pigments. The following are examples of body painting recorded throughout the world:

– Archaeological findings suggest Japanese inhabitants were already decorating their bodies in the Neolithic Jomon period (c.10,000-300 B.C.).

– In Egypt, during the time of the pharaohs, upper-class women used facepowders and other make-up, perfume, paintbrushes, and polished silver or copper mirrors.

– For thousands of years, Masai warriors used body decoration and art to express their cultural characteristics.

– In Papua, New Guinea, traditional ceremonial face paint consists of black powdered charcoal. The nose and mouth are accentuated with bright colors and white clay is used to emphasize the eyes and beard.

– The ancient Celts wore blue body paint from "woad," a type of mustard plant.

– In ancient Athens, noblewomen and courtesans applied white lead carbonate hydroxide foundation with brushes. The Roman poet Ovid wrote that the naked breasts of the Greek women were "rosy buds enhanced with a tincture of gold."

– The American Indian name "Red-Skin" came from body painting, especially among the prairie Indians.

– In India, extracts of henna plant have been used for centuries as a reddish-yellow hair dye and to decorate the hands and feet.

– In China, during the Chou dynasty of 600 B.C., members of the emperor's family wore gold and silver nail polish. Later, these colors were changed to red and black. Well-manicured nails represented the difference between the aristocrats and the working classes.

— In an ancient Peruvian grave, a mummified woman was found perfectly preserved with her light brown hair carefully combed and braided. Her legs, from knee to ankle, were painted red as was the fashion for beauties of Peru in her time. Buried along with her was her "toilet powder" (a fine powder, perhaps scented, for spreading on the body after bathing) for use in the afterlife.

The Ancient Art of Tattoo

The word tattoo comes from the Tahitian word "tatau," meaning to inflict wounds. In the centuries before modern-day tattoo needles, the tattooing process was painful and sometimes took several years to complete. Tribal tattoos were used to mark puberty, marriage, or a first successful hunt. In Polynesia, tattoo patterns were a sign of prosperity and conferred prestige. The following are additional examples of the art of tattoo throughout history:

— In 1000 B.C., Egyptian and Nubian dancers were tattooed on the thigh and pubic areas.

> "Not one great country can be named, from the polar regions in the north to New Zealand in the south, in which the aboriginals do not tattoo themselves."
> – Charles Darwin, *Voyage of the Beagle*

— Japanese aristocrats distinguished themselves with tiny tattoos near the eye. Japanese tattooists followed the lines of the muscle movements, so that when the person moved the pictures would "come alive."

— In 450 A.D., Roman soldiers gave the name "Picts" to Gallic warriors who went to battle naked in order to display their fearsome tattoos.

— The Maoris of New Zealand reserved tattooing for nobles and free people.

The First Beauty Parlors

Paleolithic statues show elaborate hair styling and braiding dating back more than 30,000 years. Early cultures worldwide used elaborate top-knots, braids, and other forms of hair styling to attract others. Roman women washed their hair with bleach made from dried nuts and acid, hoping to turn it yellow. When the Roman senate ruled that women with blond hair were to be considered prostitutes, this only increased the popularity of blond hair. In the 1700's, French hairstyles often topped four feet, and the women used wool, paste, glue, and wires to hold their hair in place.

> "For the women of my court, hairstyle remains the most important thing, the subject is inexhaustible."
> – Louis XIV

The Power of Human Beauty

> *"Fair tresses man's imperial race insnare, and Beauty draws us with a single hair".*
> *– Alexander Pope*

Of all the forms of beauty, it is the beauty of other humans that most excites us. When we see an exceptionally beautiful person, our thought process is altered, our breathing changes, our hormones surge, and our brain releases endorphins that fill our body with a sense of pleasure. Beauty may even have a positive impact on our health; one Danish/German study found that men who had survived one heart attack, after daily viewing of pictures of nude women, had a 50 percent reduction in new heart attacks.

Studies show that more attractive people are judged by others to have good personalities, be kinder and warmer, have happier marriages, have a more positive outlook on life, be more likely to live longer than average, and be more satisfied with their lives.

Beyond the way others perceive you, can sprucing up your appearance really make a difference in your life? The answer is yes. The more attractive you look, the more attention you will attract from others—and this in turn builds your sense of self-confidence. Getting attention from others in the form of admiring glances and prolonged conversations might even have a positive impact on your health. Researchers have found that massaged human infants gain weight as much as 50 percent faster than unmassaged babies, leading one to conclude that adults also physically thrive from positive attention.

Beauty and Progressive Cultures

Creative ideas and a love of physical beauty are two sides of the same coin. Historically, the areas of the world where the public has been the most attracted to the concept of physical beauty, are the areas where culture, art, science, and basic human freedoms have thrived. Conversely, the areas where physical beauty has been frowned upon or suppressed are the areas where freedom of thought, belief, and other personal liberties have been stifled.

In a sense, an obsession with personal beauty helps ignite the events that raise a society's standard of living, cure disease, and promote freedom. The statues of Athens helped create the logic of Socrates, Plato, and Aristotle. Renaissance Florence found the blend of beauty, art, science, religion, and economic activity that is still our best social model for building a successful and uplifting society.

There even appears to be a connection between the number of nude statues and paintings in an area and its economic progress. For example, the most economically vibrant region of the United States is the very tolerant and self-absorbed San Francisco Bay Area. In 2002, the per-capita income of the Bay Area was $67,000. In comparison, the second most prosperous area was Boston at $51,000. The free-living and life-loving culture of the Bay Area attracts and energizes the creative types of people who build a prosperous culture.

So the next time you reach into that jam-packed drawer of cosmetics, creams, and other concoctions, remember that you are carrying on a tradition that has been passed down through at least 75,000 years and probably much longer: the Universal Quest for Beauty in all its wonderful forms. At the same time, you are also maintaining innate human drives that produce art, science, prosperity, happiness, freedom, and civilized behavior. In revealing how the science of SRCPs is helping men and women turn back the clock, it is my hope that this book will help you reach your personal beauty goals as well.

Chapter 19

Resources

Find products at www.skinbiology.com or 1-800-405-1912
Or write to: Skin Biology – 12833 S.E. 40th Place
Bellevue, WA 98006 USA

SRCP Products for Face
- Protect & Restore Classic Cream
- Protect & Restore Cream with High Retinol and Oil of Lavender
- Protect & Restore Cream: Day Cover (with Pure Titanium Dioxide)
- CP Serum (Regular)
- Super CP Serum
- TriReduction Protect & Restore Basic
- TriReduction Protect & Restore with Retinol
- Super Cop Cream
- Super Cop Cream - 2X Extra Strength

SRCP Products for Around the Eye Area
- CP Night Eyes Premier
- CP Night Eyes Regular

Beta-Hydroxy Acids
- Exfol Cream (2% salicylic acid)
- Exfol Serum (2% salicylic acid)

SRCP Products with Hydroxy Acids built into formula
- Super CP Serum
- Super Cop Cream
- Super Cop Cream - 2X Extra Strength

SRCP Products for Scar Reduction
- Exfol Cream or Exfol Serum
- TriReduction Protect & Restore Cream
- Super CP Serum
- Super Cop Cream
- Super Cop Cream - 2X Extra Strength

SRCP Products for Body Use
- Protect & Restore Body Lotions
- Protect & Restore for Breasts, Nipples, and Décolletage
- TriReduction Protect & Restore Cream

Products for At-Risk Skin
- BioHeal
- Emu Oil-S Lipid Replenisher for Skin
- Gentle Clean Liquid Cleanser
- Gentle Clean Bar Cleanser

Biological Healing Oils / Moisturizers
- Emu Oil-S Lipid Replenisher for Skin
- Squalane
- Retinol in Squalane
- Calypso's Oil Basic (octyl palmitate/ squalane)

Body Perfumes with Plant Pheromones
- Jasmine & SB74
- Lavender & SB74
- Ylang Ylang/Nutmeg & SB74
- Patchouli & SB74
- Asian Oud & SB74
- Sandalwood & SB74
- SB74 Pheromone Only

SRCP Products for Post Sun Exposure Skin Care
- Protect & Restore Suntanning Lotion
- Protect & Restore Body Lotion for Post Tanning Skin Care

SRCP Products for Hair Growth and Condition
- Folligen Lotion
- Folligen Cream
- Folligen Spray
- Emu Oil-S for Hair
- Folligen for Blondes
- Folligen Shampoo and Conditioner

Skin Cleansers
- Gentle Clean Liquid Cleanser
- Gentle Clean Bar Cleanser

For Stronger Hydroxy Acids:
- www.skinbiology.com/resellers.com

> *See last page of book for a special introductory offer on Skin Biology Products*

Other Helpful Websites:
- www.acne.org
- www.worldhealth.net (American Academy of Anti-Aging Medicine)
- http://dermatology.cdlib.org

Other Books on Skincare, Beauty, and Health:
<u>Skincare</u>
Don't Go To The Cosmetic Counter Without Me by Paula Begoun
Wrinkle-Free by Maggie Greenwood-Robinson
Survival of the Prettiest: The Science of Beauty by Nancy Etcoff
Venus Envy: A History of Cosmetic Surgery by Elizabeth Haiken
Making the Body Beautiful: A Cultural History of Aesthetic Surgery by Sander Gilman
Inventing Beauty by Teresa Riordan
History of Beauty edited by Umberto Eco

Haircare
Hair Savers for Women by Maggie Greenwood-Robinson

Sunlight and Health
The UV Advantage by Michael F. Holick
The Healing Sun by Richard Hobday

Pheromones, Bonding, and Dating
Pure human pheromones can be purchased at
Dr. Winnifred Cutler's very informative website www.athenainstitute.com.
Also highly recommended is Dr. Cutler's book:
The Smart Women's Guide to Finding a Good Husband

Human Pheromone Sciences also sells human pheromones at a website www.naturalattraction.com

The Scent of Eros by James Vaughn Kohl and Robert T. Francoeur
The Scented Ape by Michael Stoddart
Pheromones by William Regelson
The Complete Book of Essential Oils and Aromatherapy by Valerie Ann Wormwood
Mysteries of Mating – Video – Discovery Channel Video

Diet and Supplements
Mediterranean Light by Martha Rose Shulman
The Mediterranean Diet by Nancy Harmon Jenkin
The Antioxidant Miracle by Lester Packer
The Perricone Prescription by Nicholas Perricone

Facial Exercisers
Flex Effect – www.flexeffect.com
Flex Away – www.flexawaysystem.com

If you want to use First Generation SRCPs based directly on GHK-Cu, I recommend the products from Neutrogena and ProCyte, although similar products from other companies may be effective. The Visibly Firm line by Neutrogena and Neova/Tricomin/GraftCyte lines by Procyte are supported by published proofs of efficacy.

The following are products and trademarks of the respective companies:

Neutrogena
Visibly Firm Body Lotion
Visibly Firm Night Cream
Visibly Firm Eye Cream
Visibly Firm Face Lotion SPF 20
Visibly Firm Lift Serum
Visibly Firm Night Cream
Visibly Firm Eye Treatment Concealer
Visibly Firm Moisture Makeup

Procyte
Neova Antioxidant Therapy Serum
Neova Body Therapy
Neova Cuticle Therapy
Neova Day Therapy SPF 20
Neova Eye Therapy
Neova Night Therapy
Neova Therapy Cleansing Bar
Neova Therapy Copper Moisture Mask
Neova Therapy Creme De La Copper
Neova Therapy Dual Action Lotion
Neova Therapy Mattifying Serum

Simple Solutions Ultra Copper Firming Serum
Simple Solutions Pure Copper Correcting Elixir
Simple Solutions Pure Copper Night Renewal
Simple Solutions Pure Copper Morning Dew
Simple Solutions Pure Copper Eye Repair
Simple Solutions for Men Pure Copper After Shave Moisturizer
Simple Solutions for Men Pure Copper Eye Repair

Tricomin Solution Follicle Therapy Spray
Tricomin Revitalizing Shampoo
Tricomin Restructuring Conditioner
Tricomin Conditioning Shampoo
Tricomin Deep Conditioning Treatment

GraftCyte Concentrated Spray
GraftCyte Moist Dressing
GraftCyte Post-Surgical Shampoo
GraftCyte Post-Surgical Conditioner

Complex Cu-3 Post-Laser Lotion
Complex Cu-3 Intensive Tissue Repair Creme
Complex Cu-3 Hydrating Gel
Complex Cu-3 Gentle Face Cleanser

Chapter 20

References

Chapter 9. SRCP Products for Improving the Health of Extra-Sensitive Skin 1. Zemtsov A; Gaddis M; Montalvo-Lugo VM; Australas J, "Moisturizing and cosmetic properties of Emu Oil: a pilot double-blind study," Dermatol, 1996, 37:159-61. 2. Lopez A, Sims DE, Ablett RF, Skinner RE, Leger LW, Lariviere CM, Jamieson LA, Martinez-Burnes J, Zawadzka GG, Effect of Emu Oil on auricular inflammation induced with Croton Oil in mice, Am J Vet Res 1999,60:1558-61. 3. Politis MJ, Dmytrowich A, Promotion of second intention wound healing by emu oil lotion: comparative results with furasin, polysporin and cortisone, Plast Reconstructive Surg, 1998, 102:2404-7

Chapter 10. Keeping Your Skin Young and Beautiful 1. Saxen L, Holmberg PC, Nurminen M, Kuosma E, Sauna and congenital defects, Teratology 1982, 25:309-313. 2. Paffenbarger RS, Wing AL, Hyde RT, Physical activity as an index of heart attack risk in college alumni, Am J Epidemiol 1978, 108:161-175. 3. Coastal D, The Runner, November 1984, p. 41. 4. Lopez A, Sims DE, Ablett RF, Skinner RE, Leger LW, Lariviere CM, Jamieson LA, Martinez-Burnes J, Zawadzka GG, Effect of Emu Oil on auricular inflammation induced with Croton Oil in mice, Am J Vet Res 1999,60:1558-61. 5. Politis MJ, Dmytrowich A, Promotion of second intention wound healing by emu oil lotion: comparative results with furasin, polysporin and cortisone, Plast Reconstructive Surg, 1998, 102:2404-7. 6. Traber MG, Podda M, Weber C, Thiele J, Rallis M, Packer L, Diet-derived and topically applied tocotrienols accumulate in skin and protect the tissue against ultraviolet light-induced oxidative stress, Asia Pacific J Clinical Nutrition 1997, 6:63-67 . 7. Lee A, Langer R, Shark Liver Extract Contains Inhibitors of Tumor Angiogenesis, Science 1983, 221:1185-86; Storm HM, Oh SY, Kimler BF, Norton S, Radioprotection of mice by dietary Squalene, Lipids (United States) 1993, 28:555-559. 9. Masuda A, et al, Potentiation of Anti-fungal Effect of Amphotericin B by Squalene, An Intermediate For Sterol Biosynthesis, J Antibiot 1982, 35: 230-234. 10. Garg A, Chren MM, Sands LP, Matsui MS, Marenus KD, Feingold KR, Elias PM , Psychological stress perturbs epidermal permeability barrier homeostasis: implications for the pathogenesis of stress-associated skin disorders. Arch Dermatol 2001, 137:53-9; Choi EH, Brown BE, Crumrine D, Chang S, Man MQ, Elias PM, Feingold KR, Mechanisms by which psychologic stress alters cutaneous permeability barrier homeostasis and stratum corneum integrity. J Invest Dermatol 2005, 124:587-95

Chapter 11. Improving Hair Growth and Condition with SRCPs 1. Ellis, J.A., Stebbing, M., Harrap, S.B., Genetic analysis of male pattern baldness and the 5-alpha reductase genes, J Invest Dermatol 1998; 110, 849-853. 2. Uno, H., The Histopathology of Hair Loss (Publisher: The UpJohn Company, Kalamazoo, MI) 1988. 3. The Molecular and Structural Biology of Hair (Stenn KS, Messenger AG, and Baden HP (eds). Ann NY Acad Sci, New York: New York Academy of Sciences) 1991. 4. Sugimoto Y, Lopez-Solache I, Labrie F, Luu, L, Cations inhibit specifically type I 5 alpha-reductase found in human skin, J Invest Dermatol 1995, 104:775-8

Chapter 13. Formula of Love 1. Kohl JV and Franceour RT, The Scent of Eros (Continuum Publishing) 1995; Cutler WB. Love Cycles: The Science of Intimacy, Villard (Random House), 1991, second edition 1996, Athena Institute Press; Pickart L, Formula of Love, Cosmetics & Medicine (Russia) 2005, Number 2, pages 24-33
2. Weinberg J, Porter RH: Olfaction and human neonatal behavior: clinical implications. Acta Paediatr 1998, 87:6-10; Porter RH; Winberg J, Unique salience of maternal breast odors for newborn infants. Neurosci Biobehav Rev 1999, 23:439-49; Schaal B., Coureaud G., Langlols D., Ginles C., Semon E., Perrier G. Chemical and behavioral characterization of the rabbit mammary pheromone. Nature 2003 424 (3): 68-72
3. Sobel N, Prabhakaran V, Hartley CA, Desmond JE, Glover GH, Sullivan EV, Gabrieli JD: Blind smell: brain activation induced by an undetected air-borne chemical. Brain 1999, 122:209-17
4. Hirsch A, Scentsational Sex: The Secret to Using Aroma for Arousal, 1994
5. Wyatt T.D. Pheromones and animal behavior. Communication by smell and taste. Cambridge University press. 2003
6. Umezu T; Anticonflict effects of plant-derived essential oils. Pharmacol Biochem Behav. 1999, 64:35-40; Umezu T, Behavioral effects of plant-derived essential oils in the geller type conflict test in mice, Jpn J Pharmacol. 2000, 83:150-3; de Almeida RN, Motta SC, de Brito Faturi C, Catallani B, Leite JR, Anxiolytic-like effects of rose oil inhalation on the elevated plus-maze test in rats, Pharmacol Biochem Behav. 2004 Feb;77(2):361-4;: Hongratanaworakit T, Buchbauer G. Evaluation of the harmonizing effect of ylang-ylang oil on humans after inhalation. Planta

santalol on humans after transdermal absorption, Planta Med. 2004, 70: 3-7; Heuberger E, Hongratanaworakit T, Bohm C, Weber R, Buchbauer G, Effects of chiral fragrances on human autonomic nervous system parameters and self-evaluation, Chem Senses. 2001, 26:281-92

7. Kaur M, Agarwal C, Singh RP, Guan X, Dwivedi C, Agarwal R, Skin cancer chemopreventive agent, {alpha}-santalol, induces apoptotic death of human epidermoid carcinoma A431 cells via caspase activation together with dissipation of mitochondrial membrane potential and cytochrome c release, Carcinogenesis. 2005, 26: 369-80;

Dwivedi C, Guan X, Harmsen WL, Voss AL, Goetz-Parten DE, Koopman EM, Johnson KM, Valluri HB, Matthees DP, Chemopreventive effects of alpha-santalol on skin tumor development in CD-1 and SENCAR mice, Cancer Epidemiol Biomarkers Prev, 2003, 12:151-6; Dwivedi C, Zhang Y, Sandalwood oil prevents skin tumour development in CD1 mice, Eur J Cancer Prev. 1999, 8:449-55

Chapter 14. Glowing Good Health

1. Hobday, R, The Healing Sun (Findhorn Press) 1999, 178 pages; Holick M, The UV Advantage, (Ibooks) 2003, 190 pages 2. Podda M, Traber MG, Weber C, Yan L, Packer, L : UV-Irradiation Depletes Antioxidants and Causes Oxidative Damage in a Model of Human Skin, Free Rad Biol Med 1998, 24:55-65; Morganti P, Bruno C, Guarneriz F, Cardillo A, Del Ciotto P, and Valenzanoz F; Role of topical and nutritional supplement to modify the oxidative stress. Int J Cosmet Sci 2002, 24: 331-339; Gonzalez S, Wu A, Pathak MA, Sifakis M, Goukassian DA; Oral administration of lutein modulates cell proliferation induced by acute UV-B radiation in the SHK-1 hairless mouse animal model (Abstract). The Society of Investigative Dermatology, 63rd Annual Meeting, Los Angeles, CA., 2002; Granstein RD, Faulhaber D, and Ding W; Lutein inhibits UV-B radiation-induced tissue swelling and suppression of the induction of contact hypersensitivity (CHS) in the mouse (Abstract). The Society of Investigative Dermatology, 62nd Annual Meeting, Washington D.C., 2001, p. 497; Heinrich U, Gaertner C, Wiebusch M, et al, Supplementation with beta-carotene or a similar amount of mixed carotenoids protects humans from UV-induced erythema, J. Nutrition 2003;133 :98-101; "Steenvoorden DP, Beijersbergen van Henegouwen G, Protection against UV-induced systemic immunosuppression by a single topical application of the antioxidant vitamins C and E, Int J Radiat Biol 1999 Jun;75(6):747-55; Lee J, Jiang S, Levine N, Watson RR, Carotenoid supplementation reduces erythema in human skin after simulated solar radiation exposure, Proc Soc Exp Biol Med 2000, 223:170-4; Drug and Cosmetic Industry, September 1997, pages 52-55 and December 1997, pages 40-44.

3. Marianne Berwick - (Source: Science News, Vol. 153, No. 23, June 6, 1998, p. 360

4. Ainsleigh, H. Gordon. Beneficial effects of sun exposure on cancer mortality. Preventive Medicine, 1993, 22:132-40

Garland, Cedric F, et al, Effect of sunscreens on UV radiation-induced enhancement of melanoma growth in mice. J Nat Cancer Inst, 1994, 86:798-801; Larsen, HR, Sunscreens: do they cause skin cancer, Internat J of Alternative & Complementary Med, 1994,12: 17-19; Farmer KC, Naylor MF, Sun exposure, sunscreens, and skin cancer prevention: a year-round concern, Ann Pharmacother 1996, 30:662-73; Garland, CF, et al, Could sunscreens increase melanoma risk?, Amer J Pub Health, 1992, 82: 614-615

5. Moan J, Dahlback, A, The relationship between skin cancers, solar radiation and ozone depletion, Brit. J Cancer, 1992, 65, 6:916-21

6. Stern R S, Laid N, The carcinogenic risk of treatments for severe psoriasis. Cancer 1994, 73:2759-64

7. Schlumpf M, Cotton B, Conscience M, Haller V, Steinmann B, Lichtensteiger W, In vitro and in vivo estrogenicity of UV screens, Environ Health Persp, 2001, 109:239-244

Chapter 15. Feeding your Face and Body Nutrients that Turn Back the Clock

1. Linnane AW, Zhang C, Yarovaya N, Kopsidas, Kovalenko S, Papakostopoulos HE, Graves S, Richardson, Human Aging and Global Function of Coenzyme Q-10, Ann NY Acad Sci 2002, 959: 396-411

2. Wise JA, Morin RJ, Sanderson R, Blum K , Changes in plasma carotenoid, alpha-tocopherol, and lipid peroxide levels in response to supplementation with concentrated fruit and vegetable extracts: a pilot study, Current Therapeutic Research, 1996, 57, 445-461"3. Bruce B, Spiller GA, Klevay LM, Gallagher SK, A diet high in whole and unrefined foods favorably alters lipids, antioxidant defenses, and colon function, J Am Coll Nutr, 2000 , 19,61-7

4. Gillman MW, Cupples LA, Millen BE, et al, Inverse association of dietary fat with development of ischemic stroke in men, JAMA 1997, ;278:2145-50.

5. de Lorgeril M, Salen P, Martin JL, Monjaud I, Boucher P, Mamelle N, Mediterranean dietary pattern in a randomized trial: prolonged survival and possible reduced cancer rate, Arch Intern Med. 1998 Jun 8;158(11):1181-7

6. Luigi Cornaro, Discorsi Della Vitta Sobria/Discourses on a Sober and Temperate Life 7. D'Agostino RB, 5. Elias MF, Silbershatz H, Wolf PA. Alcohol consumption and cognitive performance in the Framingham Heart Study, Am J Epidemiol. 1999, 150:580-9

Chapter 16. The Science Behind SRCPs

1. Pilgeram LO, Pickart, L Bandi, Z, Fatty acid control of fibrinogen turnover in aging and atherosclerosis, 7th International Congress of Gerontology, June 1964, pp. 451-460; Pickart L, Pilgeram LO, The role of thrombin in fibrinogen biosynthesis, Thromb Diath Haemorrh. 1967 17:358-64; Pilgeram LO, Pickart L, Control of fibrinogen biosynthesis: the role of free fatty acid, J Atheroscler Res. 1968, 8:155-66; Pickart L, Thaler MM, Fatty acids, fibrinogen and blood flow: a general mechanism for hyperfibrinogenemia and its pathologic consequences, Med Hypotheses, 1980, 6:545-57; Pickart L, Fat metabolism, the fibrinogen/fibrinolytic system and blood flow: new potentials for the pharmacological treatment of coronary heart disease, Pharmacology 1981, 23:271-80

2. A tripeptide in human plasma that increases the survival of hepatocytes and the growth of hepatoma cells. Pickart L, Ph.D.Thesis in Biochemistry, University of California, San Francisco, 1973

3. Pickart L, Thaler MM, Millard M, Effect of transition metals on recovery from plasma of the growth-modulating tripeptide glycylhistidyllysine, J Chromatogr, 1979, 175:65-73.

4. Tripeptide in human serum which prolongs survival of normal liver cells and stimulates growth in neoplastic liver, Pickart L, Thaler M, Nature New Biol,1973, 243:85-7; Pickart L, Thayer L, Thaler MM, A synthetic tripeptide which increases survival of normal liver cells, and stimulates growth in hepatoma cells, Biochem Biophys Res Commun. 1973, 54:562-6; Pickart L, Thaler, M, Purification of growth promoting peptides and proteins, and of histones, by high pressure silica gel chromatography, Prep Biochem 1975, 5:397-412; Pickart L, Thaler M, Growth modulating human plasma tripeptide: Relationship between molecular structure and DNA synthesis in hepatoma cells, FEBS Lett 1979, 104119-22; Pickart L, Lovejoy S, Biological activity of human plasma copper-binding growth factor glycyl-L-histidyl-L-lysine. Methods Enzymol 1987, 147:314-28; Pickart L, Thaler MM. Growth-modulating tripeptide (glycylhistidyllysine): association with copper and iron in plasma, and stimulation of adhesiveness and growth of hepatoma cells in culture by tripeptide-metal ion complexes. J Cell Physiol 1980, 102:129-39; Pickart L. The use of glycylhistidyllysine in culture systems. In Vitro. 1981,17:459-66; Pickart L, Freedman JH, Loker WJ, Peisach J, Perkins CM, Stenkamp RE, Weinstein B, Growth-modulating plasma tripeptide may function by facilitating copper uptake into cells, Nature. 1980, 288:715-7; Pickart L, The

biological effects and mechanism of action of the plasma tripeptide glycyl-l-histidyl-l-lysine, Lymphokines 1983, 8:425-446; Pickart L, The biological effects and mechanism of action of the plasma tripeptide glycyl-l-histidyl-l-lysine, 1983, Lymphokines 8:425-446

5. Freedman, Pickart, Weinstein, Mims, Peisach, Biochemistry, 1982, 21:4540-44; Kwa E, Bor-Sheng L, Rose N, Weinstein B, Pickart L, X-PMR studies of Cu(II) and Zn(II) interaction with glycyl-l-histidyl-l-lysine and related peptides, Peptides 1983, 8, 805-808; Perkins CM, Rose NJ, Weinstein B, Stenkamp RE, Jensen, LH, Pickart L, The structure of a copper complex of the growth factor glycyl-l-histidyl-l-lysine at 1.1 angstrom resolution, Inorg Chem Acta 1984, 82:93-99

6. Schlesinger DH, Pickart L, Thaler MM. Growth-modulating serum tripeptide is glycyl-histidyl-lysine. Experientia. 1977, 33:324-5

7. Vernon RB, Sage EH, Regulation of angiogenesis by extracellular matrix: the growth and the glue, J Hypertens Suppl 1994, 12:S145-52; Lane TF, Iruela-Arispe M, Johnson RS, Sage EH , SPARC is the source of copper-binding peptides that stimulate angiogenesis. J Cell Biol 1994, 125: 929-943.

8. Lau SJ, Sarkar B, The interaction of copper(II) and glycyl-L-histidyl-L-lysine, a growth- modulating tripeptide from plasma, Biochem J 1981 199:649-56; Laussac JP, Haran R, Sarkar B , N.m.r. and e.p.r. investigation of the interaction of copper(II) and glycyl-L-histidyl-L-lysine, a growth-modulating tripeptide from plasma, Biochem J 1983, 209:533-39

9. Freedman JH, Pickart L, Weinstein B, Mims WB, Peisach J. Structure of the Glycyl-L-histidyl-L-lysine--copper(II) complex in solution. Biochemistry. 1982, 21:4540-4

10. Pickart L, Copper Peptides for Tissue Regeneration, Specialty Chemicals, Oct. 9, 2002, 29-31.

11. Pickart. L, The use of glycylhistidyllysine in culture systems, In Vitro 1980, 17:459-66; Pickart L, Peptide and protein complexes of transition metals as modulators of cell growth; In: Chemistry and Biochemistry of Amino Acids, Peptides, and Proteins (Marcel Dekker Pub.) 1982, 75-104; Downey D, Larrabee WF, Voc i V, Pickart L. Acceleration of wound healing using glycyl-histidyl-lysine copper (II) Surg Forum 1985; 25:573-575; Pickart L., lamin: A human growth factor with multiple wound-healing properties. In: Biology of Copper Complexes (edit Sorenson J.R., Humana Press, Clifton, New Jersey, 1985) pp.273-282; Pickart, L, Copperceuticals and the skin, Cosmetics & Toiletries 2003, 118:24-28, Pickart L, Copper peptides for aging reversal, Body Language Dermatology, April 2003, 12-13; Pickart L, Skin remodeling using copper peptides, Cosmetics & Medicine (Russia) 2004, Number 2, pages 14-29, Pickart L, US Patents 4,665,054 New glycyl-L-histidyl-L-lysine-copper derivatives of improved resistance to proteolytic enzymes and better fat solubility for use in inhibiting thromboxane production and enhancing wound healing; 4,760,051 Compositions containing glycyl-l-histidyl-l-lysine copper (II) enhance the wound healing process without evoking an antigenic response, 4,810,693 Copper-glycyl-L-histidyl-L-lysine complexes enhance the healing of wounds and sores, 4,877,770 New glycyl-histidyl-lysine ester copper complex compounds with anti-inflammatory and superoxide dismutase activity useful for enhancing wound healing, 4,937,230 Method for healing wounds in horses using a copper complex of glycyl-L-histidyl-L-lysine or derivatives on the affected area, 5,164,367 Compositions for accelerating wound healing in mammals containing cupric salt or complexes with amino acid or peptide; 6,858,201 Methods for treating fingernails and toenails

12. Fish S, Katz I, Hien NR, Briden ME, Johnson JA, Patt, L, Evaluation of glycyl-1-histidyl-1-lysine copper complex in acute wound healing. Wounds 1991, 3:171-177; Counts, D, Hill E, Turner-Beatty M, Grotewiel M, Fosha-Thomas S, Pickart L. Effect of lamin on full thickness wound healing. Fed Am Soc Exp Biol 1992; A1636; Massey P, Patt L, D'Aoust JC, The effects of glycyl-l-histidyl-l-lysine copper chelate on the healing of diabetic ulcers, Wounds 4:21-28, 1992, Swaim, Bradley, Spano, McGuire and Hoffma, Evaluation of multipeptide copper complex medications on open wound healing in dogs, J Amer Ani. Hos. Assoc. 29, 519-525, 1993; Mulder, Patt, Sanders, Rosenstock, Altman, Hanley, Duncan, Enhanced healing of ulcers in patients with diabetes by topical treatment of glycyl-l-histidyl-l-lysine, Wound Rep Reg 2:259-269, 1994; Schmidt, Resser, Sims, Mullins and Smith, The combined effects of glycyl-l-histidyl-l-lysine copper (II) on the healing of linear incision wounds, Wounds 6, 62-67, 1994; Buffoni, Pino and Dal Pozzo, Effect of tripeptide-copper complexes on the process of skin wound healing and on cultured fibroblasts, Arch Int Pharmacodyn Ther 1995, 330:345-60; Swaim SF, Vaughn DM, Kincaid SA, Morrison NE, Murray SS, Woodhead MA, Hoffman C.E, Wright JC, Kammerman JR, Effect of locally injected medications on healing of pad wounds in dogs. Am J Vet Res 1996; 57: 394-399; Canapp SO Jr, Farese JP, Schultz GS, Gowda S, Ishak A.M, Swaim SF, Vangilder J, Lee-Ambrose L, Martin FG, The effect of topical tripeptide-copper complex on healing of ischemic open wounds, Vet Surg. 2003 Nov-Dec;32(6):515-23; Arul V, Gopinath D, Gomathi K, Jayakumar R. Biotinylated GHK peptide incorporated collagenous matrix: A novel biomaterial for dermal wound healing in rats. Biomed Mater Res B Appl Biomater. 2005 May;73(2):383-91

13. Pickart L, US patents 5,135,913 Skin treatment compositions comprises GHL-Cu or derivatives for improving skin health, increasing subcutaneous fat, dermal thickness and density, 5,348,943 Cosmetic and skin treatment compositions,

14. Ehrlich HP, Stimulation of skin healing in immunosuppressed rats, Symposium on Collagen and Skin Repair, Reims, Sept. 12, 1991

15. Maquart FX, Pickart L, Laurent M, Gillery P, Monboisse JC, Borel JP. Stimulation of collagen synthesis in fibroblast cultures by the tripeptide-copper complex glycyl-L-histidyl-L-lysine-Cu2+. FEBS Lett. 1988, 238:343-6; Maquart, Gillery, Monboisse, Pickart, Laurent and Borel' Glycyl-l-histidyl-l-lysine, a triplet from the a2 (I) chain of human type I collagen, stimulates collagen synthesis by fibroblast cultures; Ann. N.Y. Acad. Sci. 580:573-575, 1990; Wegrowski, Maquart, Borel, Stimulation of sulfated glycosaminoglycans by the tripeptide copper complex glycyl-l-histidyl-l-lysine copper(II), Life Sci. 51, 1049-1056, 1992; Maquart, Bellon, Chaqour, Wegrowski, Monboisse, Chastang, Birembaut and Gillery, In vivo stimulation of connective tissue accumulation by the tripeptide- copper complex glycyl-L-histidyl-L-lysine-Cu2+ in rat experimental wounds. J Clin Invest 92: 2368-76, 1993; Simeon A., Monier F. Emonard H., Gillery P., Birembaut P.. Horneback W., Maquart F.X., Expression and activation of matrix metalloproteinases in wounds: modulation by the tripeptide-copper complex glycyl-L-histidyl-L-lysine-Cu2+. J Invest Dermatol 1999; 12:957-964; Maquart F.X., Simeon A., Pasco S., Monboisse J.C., Regulation de l'activite cellulaire par la matrice extracelulaire: le concept de matrikines [Regulation of cell activity by the extracellular matrix; the concept of matrikines] French. J Soc Biol. 1999;193:423-8; Simeon A., Monier F, Emonard H, Wegrowski Y, Bellon G, Monboisse JC, Gillery P, Horneback W, Maquart FX, Fibroblast-cytokine-extracellular matrix interactions in wound repair, Curr Top Pathol. 1999;93:95-101; Simeon A., Wegrowski Y., Bontemps Y., Maquart F.X. Expression of glycosaminoglycans and small proteoglycans in wounds: modulation by the tripeptide-copper complex glycyl-L-histidyl-L-lysine-Cu(2+). J Invest Dermatol. 2000; 115:962-968; Simeon A. Emonard H., Horneback W., Maquart F.X. The tripeptide-copper complex glycyl-L-histidyl-L-lysine-Cu2+ stimulates matrix metalloproteinase-2 expression by fibroblast cultures. Life Sci. 2000; 18:2257-226

16. Aupaix F., Maquart FX, Salagnac L, Pickart L, Gillery P, Borel JP, Kalis B, Effects of the tripeptide glycyl-histidyl-lysine on healing. Clinical and biochemical correlations. J Invest Derm, 94,390,1990(abst)

17. Pickart L, US Patent US 5,118,665 New anti-oxidative and anti-inflammatory metal peptide complexes - containing glycyl-histidyl and lysine residues used to enhance or restore resistance to oxidative or inflammatory damage; Miller DM, DeSilva D, Pickart L, Aust SD. Effects of glycyl-histidyl-lysyl chelated Cu(II) on ferritin dependent lipid peroxidation, Adv Exp Med Biol 1990, 264:79-84; Coterie N, Tremolieres E, Berliner JCL, Cattier JP, Henichart JP, Redox chemistry of complexes of nickel) with some biologically important peptides in the presence of reduced

oxygen species, J Internat Bio Pharm 1992, 46:7-15; Thomas CE, The influence of medium components on Cu(2+) dependent oxidation of low-density lipoproteins and its sensitivity to superoxide dismutase. Biochem Biophys Acta 1992 1128:50-7; Vinci C., Caltabiano V, Santoro AM, Rabuazzo AM, Buscema M, Purrello R, Rizzarelli E, Copper addition prevents the inhibitory effects of interleukin 1-beta on rat pancreatic islets, Diabetologia, 1995; 38:39-45; McCormack MC, Nowak KC, Koch RJ, The effect of copper tripeptide and tretinoin on growth factor production in a serum-free fibroblast model, Arch Facial Plast Surg 2001, 3:28-32

18. Pollard JD, Quan S, Kang T, Koch RJ, Effects of copper tripeptide on the growth and expression of growth factors by normal and irradiated fibroblasts, Arch Facial Plast Surg, 2005 7:27-31

19. Raju KS, Alessandri G, Ziche M, Gullino PM, Ceruloplasmin, copper ions, and angiogenesis, J Natl Cancer Inst 1982 69(5):1183-8; Raju KS, Alessandri G, Gullino PM, Characterization of chemoattractant for endothelium induced by angiogenesis effectors. Cancer Res 1984; 44:1579-1584.

20. Unpublished observations from Hope Heart Center and Virginia Mason Research Center 1984; Manot, L, Effects du tripeptide GHK-Cu sur le Coeur isole de rat, Thesis, Universite de Reims Champagne Ardenne, 28 October 1997

21. Garcia-Sainz JA, Olivares-Reyes JA, Glycyl-histidyl-lysine interacts with the angiotensin II AT1 receptor, Peptides. 1995, 16:1203-7; Naughton BA, Naughton GK, Liu P, Zuckerman GB, Gordon AS, The influence of pancreatic hormones and diabetogenic procedures on erythropoietin production, J Surg Oncology 1982, 21:97-103

22. Poole TJ, Zetter BR, Stimulation of rat peritoneal mast cell migration by tumor derived peptides, Cancer. Res. 43, 5857-5861, 1983; Zetter B.R., Rasmussen N., Brown L. Methods of Laboratory Investigation: An In Vivo Assay for Chemoattractant Activity, Lab Invest 1985; 53:262-368; Pickart L., Downey D., Lovejoy S., Weinstein B. Gly-l-his-l-lys:copper(II) - A human plasma factor with superoxide dismutase-like and wound-healing properties, In: Superoxide and Superoxide Dismutase (Edit Rotilio, Elsevier, 1986) pages 555-558

23. Sensenbrenner M, Jaros GG, Moonen G, Mandel P, Effects of synthetic tripeptide on the differentiation of dissociated cerebral hemisphere nerve cells in culture, Neurobiology 1975, 5:207-13; Lindner G, Grosse G, Halle W, Henklein Uber die Wirkung eines synthetischen Tripeptids auf in vitro kultiviertes Nervengewebe (The effect of a synthetic tripeptide nervous tissue cultured in vitro), Z Mikrosk Anat Forsch 1979, 93:820-828; Sensenbrenner M, Jaros GG, Moonen G, Meyer BJ, Effect of conditioned media on nerve cell differentiation, Experientia. 1980, 36:660-2; Ahmed MR, Basha SH, Gopinath D, Muthusamy J, Jayakumar RJ, Initial upregulation of growth factors and inflammatory mediators during nerve regeneration in the presence of cell adhesive peptide-incorporated collagen tubes, J Peripher Nerv Syst. 2005, 10:17-30

24. Oshima H, Rochat A, Kedzia C, Kobayashi K, and Barrandon Y, Morphogenesis and renewal of hair follicles from adult multipotent stem cells, Cell, 2001, 104:233-45; Jahoda, CA, Whitehouse J, Reynolds AJ, Hole, N, Hair follicle dermal cells differentiate into adipogenic and osteogenic lineages, Exp Dermatol. 2003, 12:849-859; Lavker, RM, Sun, TT, Oshima, H, Barrandon, Y, Akiyama ,M, Ferraris, C, Chevalier, G, Favier, B, Jahoda, CA, Dhouailly, D, Panteleyev, AA, Christiano, AM, Hair follicle stem cells, J Investig Dermatol 2003, 8:28-38; Morasso MI, Tomic-Canic M, Epidermal stem cells: the cradle of epidermal determination, differentiation and wound healing, Biol Cell 2005, 97:173-83

25. Abdulghani AA, Sherr A, Shirin S, Solodkina G, Morales Tapia E, Wolf B, Gottlieb AB, Effects of creams on skin ultrastructure. DMCO 1998; 1:136-141; Abdulghani AA, Sherr A, Shirin S, Solodkina G, Morales Tapia E, Wolf B, Gottlieb AB. Studies of the effects of topical vitamin C, a copper binding cream, and melatonin cream as compared with tretinoin on the ultra structure of normal skin, J Invest Derm, 1998, 110:686(abst); Appa Y, Stephens T, Barkovic S, Finkley MB, A clinical evaluation of a copper-peptide containing liquid foundation and concealer designed for improving skin condition. Abstract P66, Amer Acad Derm Meeting February 2002; Leyden JJ, Stephens T, Finkey MB, Barkovic S, Skin care benefits of copper peptide creams, Amer Acad Derm 2002, February, Abstract P68; Leyden JJ, Stephens T, Finkey MB, Barkovic S, Skin care benefits of copper-peptide-containing eye creams., Amer Acad Derm 2002, February, Abstract P69; Sigler ML, Stephens TJ, Finkley MB, Appa Y, A clinical evaluation of a copper-peptide containing liquid foundation and cream concealer designed for improving skin condition, 60th Amer Acad Derm Meeting, New Orleans, 2002; Stephens TJ, Sigler ML, Finkley MB, Appa Y, Skin benefits of a copper peptide containing skin cream, 61th Amer Acad Derm Meeting, San Francisco, 2003; Copper Peptide and Skin, M.B. Finkley, Y. Appa, S. Bhandarkar, Cosmeceuticals and Active Cosmetic, 2nd Edition (ISBN: 0-8247-4239-7), pp 549-563

26. Pickart L. US Patents , 5,382,431 Tissue protective and regenerative compositions, 5,698,184, Compositions and methods for skin tanning and protection; 5,858,993 Starch-metal complexes for skin and hair; 5,888,522 Tissue protective and regenerative composition US 5,554,375 Tissue protective and regenerative compositions.

27. Zhai H, Poblete N, Maibach HJ, Stripped skin model to predict irritation potential of topical agents in vivo in man, Inter J Dermatol 1998, 37:386-389; Zhai H, Leow YH, Maibach HR' Human barrier recovery after acute acetone perturbation: an irritant dermatitis model, Clin Exp Derm 1998, 23:11-13; Zhai H, Leow YH, Maibach HR, Sodium laurel sulfate damaged skin in vivo in man: a water barrier repair model, Skin Res Tech 1998, 4:24-27; Zhai H, Chang YC, Singh M, Maibach HR, In vivo nickel contact dermatitis: a human model for topical therapeutics, Contact Dermatitis 1999, 40:205-208

28. Pickart, L, US Patents 5,120,831 New metal peptide complexes and derivatives used for stimulating growth of hair in warm-blooded animals, especially humans; 5,177,061 Compositions for stimulating hair growth containing cupric complexes of peptide derivatives including. glycyl-l-histidyl-l-lysine n-octyl ester; 5,214,032 New glycyl-histidyl-lysyl copper compounds used in stimulating hair growth; 5,550,183 Metal-peptide compositions and methods for stimulating hair growth; Pickart L, Skin remodeling copper peptides for improving hair growth, Cosmetics & Medicine (Russia) 2004, Number 3, pages 14-29; Pickart L, Effect of copper peptides on hair growth and condition, Body Language Dermatology 2004, Number 7, pages 20-22

29. Trachy RE, Fors TD, Pickart L, Uno H, The hair follicle-stimulating properties of peptide copper complexes. Results in C3H mice. Adv Exp Med Biol 1990, 264:79-84; Trachy RE, Fors TD, Pickart L, Uno H. The hair follicle-stimulating properties of peptide copper complexes. Results in C3H mice. Ann NY Acad Sci. 1991 Dec 26;642:468-9; Uno H and Kurata S, Chemical agents and peptides affect hair growth, J Invest Dermatol 1993 101(1 Suppl):143S-147S; Uno U, Packard S, Patt L, Dermatological Research Techniques, (CRC Press), pp-227-239, 1996; Timpe, Dumwiddie, Patt , Evaluation of Telogen Hair Follicle Stimulation Using an In Vivo Model: Results with Peptide Copper Complexes. Dermatological Research Techniques, (CRC Press), pp-241-254, 1996

30. Phototrichogram Analysis of Hair Follicle Stimulation: A pilot clinical study with a peptide-copper complex. Trachy RE, Patt, L, Duncan G, Kalis, B. Dermatological Research Techniques, (CRC Press), pp-217-226, 1996

31. Procye Corporation Press Release 1997

32. Perez-Meza, D, Leavitt, M, Trachy, R, Clinical evaluation of GraftCyte Moist Dressing on hair graft viability and quality of healing, Inter J Cos Surg 1998, 6, 80-84; Hitzig, G. Enhanced healing and growth in hair transplantation using copper peptides, Cosmetic Dermatol 2000 (June) ; 13, 18-21

33. Awa T, Nogimori K, Hairloss protection by peptide-copper complex in animal models of chemotherapy-induced alopecia. Journal Of Dermatological Science, 10, 1995, 99-104

34. Smakhtin, MY, Sever'yanova LA, Konoplya AI, Shveinov IA. Tripeptide Gly-His-Lys is a hepatotropic and immunosuppressor. Bull. Exp. Biol. Med. 2002 Jun; 133(6):586-8; Smakhtin MI, Konoplia AI, Sever'ianova LA, Sheveinov IA. Pharmacological correction of immuno-metabolic disorders with the peptide Gly-His-Lys in hepatic damage induced by tetrachloromethane. Patol Fiziol Eksp Ter. 2003 Apr-Jun; (2):19-21

35. Pickart L, US Patents 4,767,753 Copper complexes of histidyl-lysine polypeptide(s) for reducing stomach secretions, increasing stomach mucous and preventing ulcers; 5,023,237 Use of polypeptide or its copper complex for cytoprotection in treatment of intestinal and stomach ulcers, and to facilitate wound healing; 5,145,838 Methods and compositions for healing ulcers and peptide derivatives

36. Levine, Patt, Koren, An open study of PC1020 (GHK-Cu) rectal solution in treatment of distal inflammatory bowel disease, World Congress of Dermatology, October 1994; Levine, Patt, Koren,Joslin, 25th Annual Meeting of Digest Dis W, May 1995

37. Pesakova V, Novotna J, and Adam M, Effect of the tripeptide glycyl-L-histidyl-L-lysine on the proliferation and synthetic activity of chick embryo chondrocytes, Biomaterials 1995 16:911-5; Effects of the tripeptide glycyl-L-histidyl-L-lysine copper complex on osteoblastic cell spreading, attachment and phenotype, Cell Mol Biol (Noisy-le-grand) 1995 41(8):1081-91, Pohunkova H, Adam M, Reactivity and the fate of some composite bioimplants based on collagen in connective tissue, Biomaterials. 1995, 16:67-71; Pohunkova H, Stehlik J, Vachal J, Cech O, Adam M, Morphological features of bone healing under the effect of collagen-graft-glycosaminoglycan copolymer supplemented with the tripeptide Gly-His-Lys, Biomaterials 1996, 17:1567-74; Pickart L, U.S. Patent 5,059,588 Pickart Methods and compositions for healing bone using Gly His Lys: Copper

38. Pickart, US Patent 5,164,367 Method of using copper(II) containing compounds to accelerate wound healing

39. Hilfer SR, Schneck SL, Brown JW, The effect of culture conditions on cytodifferentiation of fetal mouse lung respiratory passageways. Exp Lung Res. 1986;10(2):115-36.kidney lung, Oberly TD, Murphy PJ, Steinert BW, Albrecht RM, A morphological and immunofluorescent analysis of primary guinea pig glomular cell types grown in chemically defined media, Virchows Arch [Cell Pathol] 1982, 41:145-170

Chapter 17. Copper: Your Body's Protective and Anti-Aging Metal

1. Harris ED, Copper as a cofactor and regulator of copper,zinc superoxide dismutase, J Nutr 1992, 122:636-40

2. Sorenson JR, A role for copper in mediating oxidative damage associated with degenerative disease processes seems to be more imaginary than real, Med Biol 1985;63:40-1, Sorenson (ed.), Biology of Copper Complexes Humana Press, Clifton, NJ. 1987, Sorenson JR, Copper complexes offer a physiological approach to treatment of chronic diseases, Prog Med Chem 1989; 26:437-568, Frieden E, Perspectives on copper biochemistry, Clin Physiol Biochem 1986, 4:11-19, Sorenson JR, Soderberg LS, Chidambaram MV, de la Rosa DT, Salari H, Bond K, Kearns GL, Gray RA, Epperson CE, Baker ML, Bioavailable copper complexes offer a physiologic approach to treatment of chronic diseases, Adv Exp Med Biol 1989:258:229-34.

3. Davis, C, Johnson WT, Dietary Copper Affects Azoxymethane-Induced Intestinal Tumor Formation and Protein Kinase C Isozyme Protein and mRNA Expression in Colon of Rats J Nutr 2002, 132:1018-1025,

4. Oberley LW, Leuthauser SW, Pasternack RF, Oberley TD, Schutt L, Sorenson JR, Anticancer activity of metal compounds with superoxide dismutase activity, Agents Actions 1984, 15:535-8

5. Greene FL, Lamb LS, Barwick M, Pappas NJ, Effect of dietary copper on colonic tumor production and aortic integrity in the rat J Surg Res, 1987, 42:503-12; Narayanan VS, Fitch CA and Levenson CW, Tumor suppressor protein p53 mRNA and subcellular localization are altered by changes in cellular copper in human Hep G2 cells, J Nutr 2001, 131:1427-32

6. Klevay LM, Hypertension in rats due to copper deficiency. Nutr. Rep. Int. 1987, 35:999-1005; Klevay LM, Halas ES, The effects of dietary copper deficiency and psychological stress on blood pressure in rats, Physiol Behav 1991, 49:309-14; levay LM, Trace elements, atherosclerosis, and abdominal aneurysms, Ann N Y Acad Sci 1996, 800:239-42; Klevay LM, Cardiovascular disease from copper deficiency--a history, J Nutr 2000, 130:489S-492S; Klevay LM, Dietary copper and risk of coronary heart disease, Am J Clin Nutr 2000, 71:1213-4; Klevay LM, Extra dietary copper inhibits LDL oxidation, Am J Clin Nutr 2002, 76:687-8; Klevay L, Ischemic heart disease as deficiency disease, Cell Mol Biol (Noisy-le-grand) 2004, 50:877-84;

7. Institute of Medicine. Dietary reference intakes for vitamin A, vitamin K, boron, chromium, copper, iodine, iron, manganese, molybdenum, nickel, silicon, vanadium, and zinc. Washington, D.C.: National Academy Press. 2001

8. Rock E, Mazur A, O'connor JM, Bonham MP, Rayssiguier Y, Strain JJ, The effect of copper supplementation on red blood cell oxidizability and plasma antioxidants in middle-aged healthy volunteers, Free Radic Biol Med. 2000 , 28:324-9

9. Greene FL, Lamb LS, Barwick M, Pappas NJ, Effect of dietary copper on colonic tumor production and aortic integrity in the rat .J Surg Res, 1987, 42:503-12

10. Bala S, Failla ML, Copper deficiency reversibly impairs DNA synthesis in activated T lymphocytes by limiting interleukin 2 activity. Proc Natl Acad Sci U S A, 1992, 89:6794-7

11. Heresi G, Castillo-Duran C, Munoz C, Arevalo M, & Schlesinger L, Phagocytosis and immunoglobulin levels in hypocupremic infants. Nutr Res, 1985, 5: 1327-1334

12. Kelley DS, Daudu PA, Taylor PC, Mackey BE, Turnlund JR, Effects of low-copper diets on human immune response, Am J Clin Nutr 1995, 62:412-6

13. Balu U, Failla ML, Copper status and function of neutrophils are reversibly depressed in marginally and severely copper deficient rats, J Nutr 1990,120:1700-1709; Bala S, Failla ML, Copper deficiency reversibly impairs DNA synthesis in activated T lymphocytes by limiting interleukin 2 activity, Proc Natl Acad Sci U S A 1992, 89:6794-7

14. Sorenson JR, Hangarter W, Treatment of rheumatoid and degenerative diseases with copper complexes: A review with emphasis on copper-salicylate. Inflammation, 1977;2:217-238; Sorenson JR, Evaluation of copper complexes as potential anti-arthritic drugs, J Pharm Pharmacol. 1977, 29:450-2; Dollwet and Sorenson, Historic uses of copper compounds in medicine, Trace Elements in Medicine, Vol. 2, No. 2, 1985, pp 80-87; Sorenson JR, Antiinflammatory, analgesic, and antiulcer activities of copper complexes suggest their use in a physiologic approach to treatment of arthritic diseases, Basic Life Sci. 1988;49:591-4.

15. Dollwet HH, Sorenson JR, Roles of copper in bone maintenance and healing, Biol Trace Elem Res 1988, 18:39-48; Conlan D, Korula R, Tallentire D, Serum copper levels in elderly patients with femoral-neck fractures. Altern Med Rev 1990, 19:212-214; Jonas J, Burns J, Abel, EW, Cresswell MJ, Strain,JJ, Paterson CR, Impaired mechanical strength of bone in experimental copper deficiency, Ann Nutr Metab 1993, 37:245-252; Baker A, Harvey L, Majask-Newman, G, Fairweather-Tait, S, Flynn A, Cashman K, Effect of dietary copper intakes on biochemical markers of bone metabolism in healthy adult males, Eur J Clin Nutr 1999, 53:408-412

16. Sorenson JR, Ramakrishna K, Rolniak TM Antiulcer activities of D-penicillamine copper complexes. Agents Actions. 1982, 12:408-11; Alzuet G, Ferrer S, Borras J, Sorenson JR, Anticonvulsant properties of copper acetazolamide complexes .J Inorg Biochem. 1994 Aug 1;55(2):147-51; Morgant G, Dung NH, Daran JC, Viossat B, Labouze X, Roch-Arveiller M, Greenaway FT, Cordes W, Sorenson JR Low-temperature crystal

structures of tetrakis-mu-3,5-diisopropylsalicylatobis-dimethylformamido-dicopper(II) and tetrakis-mu-3,5-diisopropylsalicylatobis-diethyletheratodicopper(II) and their role in modulating polymorphonuclear leukocyte activity in overcoming seizures. J Inorg Biochem. 2000 Jul 15;81(1-2):11-22; Lemoine P, Viossat B, Morgant G, Greenaway FT, Tomas A, Dung NH, Sorenson JR. Synthesis, crystal structure, EPR properties, and anti-convulsant activities of binuclear and mononuclear 1,10-phenanthroline and salicylate ternary copper(II) complexes, J Inorg Biochem 2002, 89:18-28; Viossat B, Greenaway FT, Morgant G, Daran JC, Dung NH, Sorenson JR, Low-temperature (180 K) crystal structures of tetrakis-mu-(niflumato)di(aqua)-dicopper(II) N,N-dimethylformamide and N,N-dimethylacetamide solvates, their EPR properties, and anticonvulsant activities of these and other ternary binuclear copper(II)niflumate complexes, J Inorg Biochem 2005, 99:355-67 17. Morten MS, Elwood PC, Abernethy M, Trace elements in water and congenital malformations of the central nervous system in South Wales, Br J Prev Soc Med 1976, 30:36-39; Ebbs JH, Tisdall FF, Scott WA, The influence of prenatal mother and child, J Nutr 1991, 22:515-526; Keen CL, Uriu-Hare JY, Hawk SN, Jankowski MA, Daston GP, Kwik-Uribe CL, Rucker RB, Effect of copper deficiency on prenatal development and pregnancy outcome, Am J Clin Nutr 1998, 67:1003S-1011S; Lonnerdal B, Copper nutrition during infancy and childhood, Am J Clin Nutr 1998, 67:1046S-1053S; Hawk SN, Lanoue L, Keen CL, Kwik-Uribe CL, Rucker RB, Uriu-Adams JY, Copper-deficient rat embryos are characterized by low superoxide dismutase activity and elevated superoxide anions, Biol Reprod. 2003 Mar;68(3):896-903; Penland JG, Prohaska JR, Abnormal motor function persists following recovery from perinatal copper deficiency in rats, J Nutr 2004, 134:1984-8;

18. Saari, J.T., Bode A.N., Dahlen G.W. Defects of copper deficiency on rats are modified by dietary treatments that affect glycation. 1995; 125: 2925-2934

19. Bhathena SJ, Recant L, Voyles NR, Timmers KI, Reiser S, Smith JC, Powell AS, Decreased plasma enkephalins in copper deficiency in man, Am J Clin Nutr. 1986, 43:42-6; Okuyama S, Hashimoto S, Aihara H, Willingham WM, Sorenson JR, Copper complexes of non-steroidal antiinflammatory agents: analgesic activity and possible opioid receptor activation, Agents Actions 1987, 21:130-44

20. Klevay LM, Christopherson DM, Copper deficiency halves serum dehydroepiandrosterone in rats, J Trace Elem Med Biol, 2000 14:143-5

Index

A

abrasion *31*
acid mantle *90*
acne *94*
acne scars *69*
age spots *65*
aging reversal *9*
alien chemicals *12*
alpha hydroxy acids *27. See also 69*
alpha lipoic acid *150*
antioxidants *31*
arginine/ornithine *150*
artificial implants *18*
artificial methods *18*
ascorbic acid. *See Vitamin C*
astringents *93*
attraction *126*

B

baby fat *21. See also 103*
bath, bathing *91*
beauty *176*
bedsores *79*
beta hydroxy acids *27. See also 69*
biological healing oils *28*
blackheads *91. See also 94*
blemish removal *64*
blond hair, green out *109*
blood circulation *158*
body perfumes *132*
bonding *127*
bone healing *166*
botulinum toxin *18*
bovine collagen *18*
breast lift *57*
burns, radiation *85*
burns, thermal *85*

C

calcium *150*
chemical peels *73*
chemoattraction *158*
choline / inositol *150*
chondroitin sulfate *150*
clarifying shampoos *114*
coenzyme Q10, CoQ-10 *98*
collagen *95. See also 106, 156*
color cosmetics *13. See also 33*
comedos *82*
conditioners *115*
contact dermatitis *86*
copper and disease *170*
copper, daily *150. See also 169*
copper, healing *168*
copper, love *174*
cortisol *174*
cortisone *163*
cosmetic moisturizers *96*

D

dermabrasion *21. See also 31, 50*
dermatitis *86*
DHEA *143. See also 150, 174*
DHT (dihydrotestosterone) *102*
diabetes *85*
diet *144*
dietary fiber *148*
DMAE *35*
DNA *157*
dry skin *84*

E

eczema *83*
elastin *40*
emu oil *88. See also 97*
exercise *95*
exfoliating hydroxy acids *27*
expensive perfumes *128*

E

eye area *42*
eyebrows *122*
eyelashes *122*
eyelids *42*. See also *94*

F

fiber *145*
fibroblasts *54*
folic acid *149*
fragile, sensitive skin *79*
free radicals *80, 81*. See also *140*

G

gamma linolenic acid *150*
GHK-Cu *24*. See also *155*
ginkgo biloba *150*
glow *11*
glucosamine *150*
glycyl-histidyl-lysine *155*
GraftCyte *106*. See also *165*
grape seed extract *150*

H

hair, brushing *117*
hair, color *114*
hair, damage *114*
hair, follicles *159*
hair, gray *113*
hair, growth *117*
hair, hormone shifts *104*
hair, length *113*
hair, loss *104*
hair, permanents *119*
hair, relaxers *120*
hair, removal *121*
hair, straightening *120*
hair, thinning *104*
hair transplantation *165*
hands *95*
heating lights *57*
HIV/AIDS skin problems *87*
hyaluronic acid *38*
hydrogen peroxide *82*

I

immune deficient *172*
immune-compromised *87*
inflammation *163*
infra-red machines *18*
intestinal healing *166*

J

jewelry *177*
junk science *13*

K

keratin *112*

L

lactic acid *69*
laser resurfacing *16*. See also *18, 21*
lipids *90*
lips *99*
liver, restore *166*
Long Hair Clinics *102*
loose, sagging skin *53*
lutein *98*
lycopene *98*

M

magnesium *150*
make-up *35*. See also *42, 75*
melanin *106*
melatonin *150*
methods of Skin Renewal *18*
microwaves *18*
minoxidil *108*
Models and Actors *75*
moisturizers *18*
moles *72*
moral need *176*
MSM (methylsulfonylmethane) *150*

N

N-acetyl-carnitine *150*
nerve outgrowth *158*
nerve paralyzers *18*
neuropeptides *12*

O

omega fatty acids *145*. See also *149, 150*

P

pheromones *125*
photodamage *24*
phytonutrients *146*
pitted scars *69*
plant extracts, toxic *13*
pore cleansing *59*
pore size *59*

P

pores, tighten 59
pregnant, pregnancy 173
propecia 100
psoriasis 87

R

remodeling, skin 19
retinoic acid 30
retinol 30
reverse aging 9
rosacea 74

S

sagging skin 53
salicylic acid 69
saunas 93
saw palmetto oil 150
scalp damage 106
scars 62-72
second-generation SRCPs 25
shampoo 114
shaving 121
shower 91
silicone injections 17
Sjorgren's Syndrome 84
skin allergies 85
skin barrier damage 80
skin fillers 18. *See also* 39
skin firmness 53, 54
skin products 37
skin remodeling copper-peptides (SRCPs) 23
skin tags 70
skin ulcers 82
soap pH 92
soy isoflavones 150
squalane 98
stem cells 159
Stepford Wives 12
strength of SRCPs in Skin Biology products 34
stress 9,10. *See also* 75, 99, 134
stretch marks 71
subcutaneous fat 21
sulfur donor 103
sun damage 71
sunblockers 140
sunlight health 137
sunscreens, chemical 140
suntanning 137
supplements 150

T

terminal hair follicles 159
TGF-ß-1 (transforming growth factor) 21
tissue repair 166
tocotrienols 98
toners 93
toothpick trick for scars 65
trans-fats 145
Tricomin 106. *See also* 165

U

unnatural methods 18

V

vegetable extracts 146
vellus hair follicles 159
vitamin C 30
vitamins 149

W

wheelchairs 79. *See also* 81
whiteheads 82
wine 152
wound healing 25
wrinkles 39, 40

X

X-ray, acne 17

Z

zinc 150

Skin Biology

SECOND GENERATION SRCPs

50% Introductory Offer

Use this page for a 50% discount on the purchase of up to $100 of Skin Biology Products

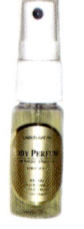

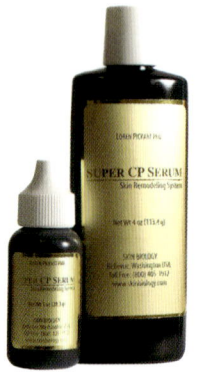

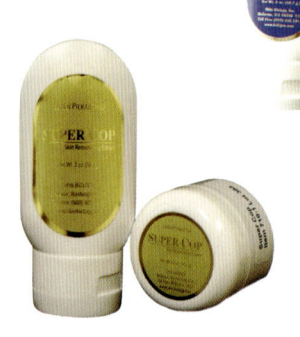

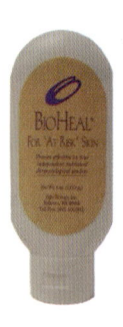

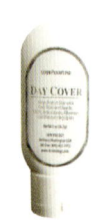

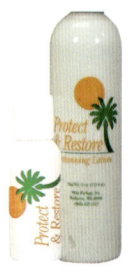

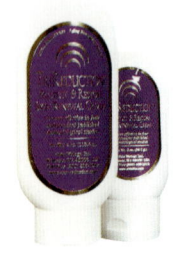

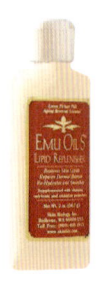

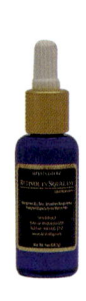

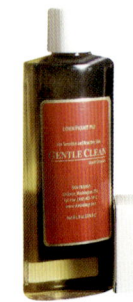

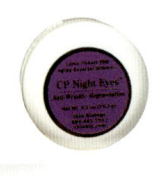

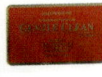

— Log on to www.skinbiology.com to order —

CUT HERE

This coupon is good for one order only. Products must be ordered directly from Skin Biology. Offer does not include shipping and handling.